OCCUPATIONAL HAZARDS IN DENTISTRY

Occupational Hazards in Dentistry

Harriet S. Goldman, D.D.S., M.P.H., F.A.C.D.
Associate Professor of Oral Medicine
Director, Hospital Dentistry and Special Patient Care
New York University College of Dentistry
New York, New York

Kenton S. Hartman, D.D.S., M.S.D.
Chairman, Department of Oral Pathology
Armed Forces Institute of Pathology
Washington, D.C.

Jacqueline Messite, M.D.
Regional Program Consultant
National Institute for Occupational Safety and Health
New York, New York

YEAR BOOK MEDICAL PUBLISHERS, INC.
CHICAGO

0   9   8   7   6   5   4   3   2   1

Library of Congress Cataloging in Publication Data

Main entry under title:
Occupational Hazards in Dentistry
   1. Dental offices—Hygienic aspects.   2. Dental personnel—Diseases and
hygiene.   3. Environmentally induced diseases.   I. Goldman, Harriet S.
II. Hartman, Kenton S.   III. Messite, Jacqueline   DNLM: 1. Dentistry.
2. Occupational diseases—Prevention and control.   3. Accidents,
Occupational—Prevention and control. WA 412 D414
RK3.025 1984   616.9'803   84-3501
ISBN 0-8151-3755-9

Sponsoring editor: Diana L. McAninch
Editing supervisor: Frances M. Perveiler
Copyeditor: Kareen Snider
Production project manager: Dorothy J. Mulligan
Proofroom supervisor: Shirley E. Taylor

For Michael L. B. Kaplan, Esq., Marguerite Hartman, R.N., and Dauber Telsey, D.D.S.—husbands and wife who didn't begrudge us the time to do this important work.

Contributors

ARDEN G. CHRISTEN, D.D.S., M.S.D., M.A., Chairman, Department of Preventive Dentistry, Indiana University School of Dentistry, Indianapolis, Indiana

ROBERT L. COOLEY, D.M.D., M.S., Dental Investigation Service, USAF School of Aerospace Medicine (AFSC), Brooks AFB, Texas

LARRY J. CRABB, D.D.S., Department of Family Practice, University of Iowa College of Dentistry, Iowa City, Iowa

HARRIET S. GOLDMAN, D.D.S., M.P.H., F.A.C.D., Associate Professor of Oral Medicine, Director, Hospital Dentistry and Special Patient Care, New York University College of Dentistry, New York, New York

WILLIAM GREENFIELD, D.D.S., Associate Dean for Hospital and Extramural Affairs, Professor of Oral and Maxillofacial Surgery, New York University College of Dentistry, New York, New York

NORMAN O. HARRIS, D.D.S., M.S.D., F.A.C.D., Department of Community Dentistry, The University of Texas Dental School at San Antonio, San Antonio, Texas

KENTON S. HARTMAN, D.D.S., M.S.D., Chairman, Department of Oral Pathology, Armed Forces Institute of Pathology, Washington, D.C.

OLGA A.C. IBSEN, R.D.H., M.S., Associate Clinical Professor, Columbia University, Columbia Presbyterian Medical Center, New York, New York

JACQUELINE MESSITE, M.D., Regional Program Consultant, National Institute for Occupational Safety and Health, New York, New York

MAURICE H. MILLER, PH.D., Professor, Program of Speech Pathology and Audiology, Department of Communications, School of Education, Health, Nursing and Arts Professions, New York University, New York, New York

JEANNE M. STELLMAN, PH.D., Associate Professor, Division of Health Administration, School of Public Health, Columbia University, and Executive Director, Women's Occupational Health Resource Center (at Columbia), New York, New York

Contents

Foreword

WORK IS A MAJOR DETERMINANT of our income, style of life, social interactions, and health. We are increasingly aware that all work is characterized by certain stresses. In the not-too-distant past, those occupations with major, dramatic impacts on health, e.g., mining, construction, and lumbering, among others, were highlighted because of the very great risks imposed upon workers. During the last 20 to 30 years, epidemiologists have teased out associations between risk factors and their effects on our health; one of these factors has been occupation. The future will undoubtedly bring a host of publications describing the particular health hazards of any given profession.

As a forerunner in this regard, this book contains a series of chapters relating to the broad concerns of the dentist in his/her occupational environment. Chapter 1, by Dr. Jacqueline Messite, is an overview. Here we learn that there are approximately 125,000 dentists practicing in the United States, and that over 93% of these employ at least one other person, with one third employing four or more auxiliary persons. Potential hazards to dentists include infection from airborne and bloodborne organisms, disorders caused by chemical agents in the form of waste anesthetic agents and airborne particulates, mercury, ethylene oxide, beryllium, physical skeletal disorders, and general stress. Chapter 2 on aerosol hazards by Dr. Robert L. Cooley delineates the sources of aerosols and preventive measures that can be used. While it is not clear that potential hazards are realized in practice, a survey of possible sources is impressive. Dr. Kenton S. Hartman discusses infectious and communicable diseases, including fungal, viral, and microbial infections. He describes practical ways for dentists to exercise preventive measures.

The dangers of mercury to dentists have been well documented. Pathways of entry into the body are through inhalation of vapors and direct absorption into the tissues from mercury compounds that penetrate the skin. The author, Dr. Harriet S. Goldman, describes the nature of the problem and the methods for intervention in Chapter 4.

Physical, chemical, and thermal injuries are treated by Dr. Robert L. Cooley, and hearing conservation programs for dentists are described by

Dr. Maurice H. Miller. The general subject of stress and distress in the dental office is described by Dr. Arden G. Christen. Proper positioning and work habits are important aspects of ergonomics as discussed by Dr. Norman Harris and Dr. Larry Crabb. A review of radiation hygiene practices in the dental office is presented by Olga Ibsen, R.D.H., and Dr. William Greenfield enlightens us with his discussion of anesthetic gas hazards in the dental environment.

This is a book for those interested in occupational health and trends for the future. If we only had a series of volumes describing the potential hazards of each of our professions, those practicing in this field could have easy access to understanding the environment and planning preventive interventions. Such an approach is closely related to the current emphasis on "right to know" laws. It has taken a long time, but we are finally focusing on the health risks of specific occupations. The authors of this volume are to be applauded.

MORTON CORN, M.D.
DIRECTOR
DEPARTMENT OF ENVIRONMENTAL HEALTH SCIENCES
SCHOOL OF PUBLIC HEALTH
JOHNS HOPKINS UNIVERSITY
BALTIMORE, MARYLAND

Preface

DENTAL EDUCATION has been remiss in adequately preparing dentists and auxiliary personnel to recognize and avoid many of the occupational hazards in the dental environment. Our general environment contains many health hazards that can kill, injure, and disable people. In fact, the National Institute for Occupational Safety and Health estimates that 100,000 Americans die annually from occupationally related illnesses, and another 400,000 new cases of occupationally related diseases occur each year.

During the past decade, numerous literature and media reports about health hazards in the dental setting have undoubtedly helped to make dental personnel more aware of potential health hazards in their workplace. In the past, the dental curriculum has been primarily concerned with the preservation of health and well-being of the patients, and inadequate attention was paid to the health of the dental provider. There was only minimal consideration given to the potentially hazardous environment for dental personnel and the untoward effects it could have upon their health. Dentistry as a whole is now more aware of these potential health hazards and how to implement proper protective measures.

This handbook is designed to acquaint dental students, dentists, dental assistants, and dental hygienists with many of the environmental problems they may encounter in a dental office. Another objective is to describe symptoms of dental occupationally related diseases and to suggest means for their prevention and control.

Multiple contributors have worked together to encompass the entire spectrum of dental occupational hazards. The compilation of their experiences has resulted in a ready reference that has everyday practical significance and suggests measures to avoid damaging injuries; exposure to infectious diseases; mercury toxicity; anesthetic, noise, and radiation hazards; ergonomic considerations; and management of stress-related problems. In addition, appendices are provided that list federal and state agencies to contact for additional information or guidelines.

Christen and Harris have so aptly stated that "as dentists and auxiliaries, we spend half of our waking hours at the office. Let us learn to work in safety, comfort, and tranquility."

HARRIET S. GOLDMAN, D.D.S., M.P.H., F.A.C.D.
KENTON S. HARTMAN, D.D.S., M.S.D.
JACQUELINE MESSITE, M.D.

Chapter 1

Occupational Safety and Health in the Dental Workplace

Jacqueline Messite, M.D.

OCCUPATIONAL SAFETY AND HEALTH has been a matter for concern since people began working. Reference to harmful effects of work exposures to chemicals can be found in the writings of Hippocrates and in other Greek and Roman literature. As early as the fourth century B.C., physicians were aware that chemicals in the mines were causing fatalities among the workers. Ancient Roman slaves laboring in mercury mines devised bladder skin masks in their feeble attempt to avoid inhaling the fumes. In the 17th century, Bernardino Ramazzini published the first comprehensive treatise on occupational diseases *De Morbis Artificium Diatriba* ("The Discourse on the Diseases of Workmen"), and recommended that doctors inquire about a patient's occupation when taking a history. In 1775, Percival Pott, an English surgeon, noted numerous cases of scrotal cancer among chimney sweeps exposed to coal tar. In the United States, occupational health and safety were not addressed to any extent until the early 20th century. One of the pioneers in American occupational health and safety was Dr. Alice Hamilton. Her autobiography, *Exploring the Dangerous Trades*, relating her experiences in investigating cases of occupational diseases in this country is a classic in this field. The status of occupational safety and health in American industry in the early part of this century is vividly described in her book.

Reports concerning the health and safety of dentists have appeared in the literature since the late 1920s. The earliest report of the mortality experience of persons engaged in the profession of dentistry dates from the late 1920s with the publication of the *Registrar General's Decennial Supplement, England and Wales, Occupational Mortality (1927)*. In that publication, the mortality experience of dentists was for the first time described separately from other health professionals. Relating the dentists of 1920 to 1922 to the census of 1921, the report indicates that the compara-

1

tive mortality was lower for dentists than for medical practitioners. These rates were 910 for dentists, compared with 1,021 for physicians.

Subsequent decennial reports from England and Wales in 1938, 1958, and 1971 have disclosed similar findings indicating that the mortality experience of dentists is the same or better than that of the general population or their professional peers. However, these reports noted certain causes of death to be in excess, namely cardiovascular diseases and suicide.

The American Dental Association (ADA) published the results of a study of 3,707 reported deaths among dentists between 1951 and 1954. The source of the information was death certificates forwarded to the ADA in a cooperative study with a majority of the state health departments. Data were reported only for white male dentists and as percentages adjusted for differences between the age distributions of living dentists and the 1952 white male population. As with the reports from England and Wales, significantly higher percentages of deaths were recorded for diseases of the circulatory system and suicide, although the latter was not statistically significant. Excess of deaths from diseases of the circulatory system in dentists was also found in similar studies by the ADA covering periods 1955 to 1960 and 1961 to 1966.

These excesses were not found in more recent studies, however. Orner and Breslin, in a study sponsored by the National Institute for Occupational Safety and Health (NIOSH) at Temple University's School of Dentistry, reviewed the mortality experience between 1960 and 1965 of a cohort of 102,726 dentists, of which 8,945 died during the period of study. Using the mortality data for the United States white male population, their findings indicated that the Standardized Mortality Ratio (SMR) for dentists for all causes was less than for the general male population (0.71), with significant deficits for nearly all causes. The authors concluded that there are no excesses of cancer among dentists in general and that the suicide rate, purportedly a higher risk among dentists, is approximately equal to that of the general population.

Similarly, the Bureau of Economic Research and Statistics of the ADA received death certificates from 31 state health departments for 4,190 dentists dying between 1968 and 1972. A comprehensive analysis of the data indicated that in most instances the percentage of dentists dying from specified causes was very similar to that of the white male population in the same age categories. The most frequent causes of death for both groups were diseases of the circulatory system, neoplasms, and diseases of the nervous system and sense organs. Diseases of the circulatory system accounted for 51.74% among dentists and 51.71% of the deaths among white males. The corresponding figures for neoplasms were 17.70% and 17.73%, and for diseases of nervous system and sense organs, 9.03% and 9.07%.

Accidents, poisonings (no details were given as to type), and violence were the leading causes of death for dentists under age 50 years, and diseases of the circulatory system and neoplasms were leading causes for those 55 years and older.

It is difficult to relate the various mortality studies to each other because of the many different approaches that have been taken in doing the studies and the varying ways of reporting the findings. However, all have one common finding, and that is that dentists generally have a more favorable overall mortality experience than the general population and a lower mortality than their professional peers.

The practice of dentistry today is not categorized as a high-risk occupation, and the degree of exposure to chemical and physical agents usually is not of a life-threatening magnitude. It is not surprising therefore, that the many mortality studies that have been done on dentists through the years have not disclosed any overall increased mortality.

However, the concerns for occupational safety and health of dentists would be masked if one were only to look at mortality data. The type and degree of exposures in the dental offices and clinics have the potential for increased morbidity. Furthermore, studies of dentists as a general group may also mask morbidity experience, because dentists in different specialties and practices have different occupational exposures. For example, while mercury exposure would be more common in the office of general practitioners, it is less likely to be present in offices of orthodontists. The use of anesthetic gases with the resultant potential for exposure to waste gases is not usual in offices of general practitioners or orthodontists, but is common in offices of oral surgeons and periodontists. Furthermore, if an office has an associated dental laboratory, exposures to multiple substances such as acrylics and various solvents could be part of the exposure of all persons working in the office. Therefore, it is more meaningful to study the morbidity experience of dentists and dental workers in similar specialties with similar types of work practices and operations.

Dentists and dental health professionals constitute a sizable occupational group at risk to multiple exposure. The total number of dentists in the United States in 1979 (including all 50 states, territories, and outlying areas) was 124,952, with an additional 6,214 employed in the Armed Forces and other federal installations. An ADA survey of dental practices in 1977 indicated that over 93% of the dentists employed at least one auxiliary person and 33% reported employing four or more auxiliary persons including hygienists, chair-side assistants, laboratory technicians, and related office personnel.

In the practice of dentistry, dentists and auxiliary personnel can be exposed to chemical, physical, and biologic agents as well as to stressful environments. The degree of exposure to these agents is generally below the present permissible Occupational Safety and Health Administration (OSHA) limits, but exposures in excess of acceptable limits have been found in a number of dental offices and clinics. Of the 31 health hazard evaluations involving dental offices requested of NIOSH between 1976 and 1981, excessive exposures were found in 16 (51.6%). Four of these involved exposure to mercury and 12 to waste anesthetic gases, particularly nitrous oxide. While these evaluations represent a biased sample in that they were the offices or clinics for which health hazard evaluations were requested because excessive exposures were suspected to exist, it is reasonable to assume that similar conditions are present and unrecognized in many other dental facilities. Table 1–1 is a list of the major occupational health and safety considerations in this field.

Infections

Outbreaks of various transmissible diseases in the general population are a constant reminder of the perpetual need for effective measures to prevent disease transmission during dental treatment. The potential for infection in the dental operatory is recognized, as is the ease of transmittal.

Although protection of the patient is an obvious priority, available data indicate that dental personnel are also vulnerable to cross infection. For example, one outbreak of *Mycoplasma pneumoniae* infection was reported among prosthodontic laboratory personnel. Investigation revealed that transmission of the organism was caused by a fine-particle aerosol generated from abrasive grinding of contaminated dentures. Furthermore, approximately one person in 70 carries herpes simplex in his/her saliva that may affect unprotected eyes or enter small, unprotected lesions on fingers.

A research project completed at the Ohio State University dental hygiene clinic (Autio and coworkers) revealed eight pathogenic organisms indigenous to human oral flora that transfer significantly from the patient to the operator and from the operator to the environment, which includes the handles of the sink and the switches of the dental chair unit. Recognized procedures of cleanliness, disinfection, and sterilization should be routine in dental operatories. During high-speed operative procedures, dentists can be exposed to microbial aerosols consisting of carious dental pulp and water droplets contaminated with organisms from the patient's saliva. Travaglini and coworkers evaluated the organisms carried in the aerosol by using a disposable paper face mask with a plastic eye shield to catch droplets ejected from the patient's mouth. The pretest cultures of the patients' masks, dentist's mask, burs, and handpieces were essentially uncontaminated. After each operation, the face masks were examined. At an average

TABLE 1–1.—OCCUPATIONAL HEALTH AND SAFETY CONSIDERATIONS
FOR DENTISTS AND DENTAL HEALTH PERSONNEL

Infections
  Airborne organisms (direct exposure from patient contact or released in high-speed
  drilling)
    Bacteria
    Viruses
  Blood-borne organisms
    Hepatitis B virus
    Acquired immune deficiency syndrome
Disorders caused by the following:
  Chemical agents
    Waste anesthetic gases (nitrous oxide, halothane, other chlorinated compounds, etc.)
    Airborne particulates
      Mineral dusts released in high-speed drilling
      Asbestos and other fibrous dusts (buffing compounds)
    Acrylics (methacrylate and others)
    Ethylene oxide (sterilization)
    Mercury
    Beryllium
  Physical agents
    Ionizing radiation (x-rays)
    Ultraviolet light
    Noise (high-speed handpiece)
    Ultrasound
  Dermatitis
    Contact (soaps, detergents)
    Irritation (soaps, detergents, bonding compounds, zinc chloride, fluorides)
    Allergic dermatitis (acrylics, mercury, antibiotics, benzocaine, procaine, benzoyl
      peroxides)
  Musculoskeletal disorders: Ergonomic factors (positional and postural)
  Injuries
    Back injuries (incorrect work posture)
    Eye injuries (high-speed drilling, spray from cavitron, scaling, rotating instruments,
      polishing pastes)
  Stress
    Interpersonal relationships (dentist-staff-patients)
    Office routine (appointment scheduling [overbooking], broken appointments)
    Procedural stresses (long operatory procedures, working in small, restricted areas of the
      mouth, lack of patient cooperation, apprehensive patients)

working distance of 15 to 20 in., there appeared to be no zone of safety from the organism-bearing droplets. In all 20 patients studied, a significant number of colonies were plated. Alpha streptococcus was the largest component of the oral flora, but other organisms found include beta and gamma streptococcus, *Bacillus subtilis*, *Staphylococcus aureus*, and diphtheroids. This study demonstrated that both the dentist and the patient are at risk of being contaminated with living organisms from the oral cavity during routine operative procedures. The authors noticed that simple protective devices such as disposable masks with a plastic eye shield act as an effective mechanical barrier to the propelled organism-bearing droplets.

Three of the infections of most concern to the dentist and the dental staff are herpes, hepatitis, and acquired immune deficiency syndrome (AIDS).

Herpes

Herpes simplex virus (HSV) is responsible for a variety of clinical syndromes affecting the skin, mucous membranes, and nervous system. Infections with HSV occur as either primary or recurrent herpetic stomatitis. Dental personnel are at particular risk from primary herpetic infection because of frequent exposure. In addition, a study by Brooks and coworkers of dentists and dental students at the University of Michigan School of Dentistry showed that 43% of those studied had no evidence of HSV disease either by history or by serologic studies and were therefore at more risk of contacting the virus than the general adult population when they were treating patients with active lesions. Because herpetic lesions, particularly of the eye and finger, can present serious problems for the practicing dentist, it is important that the nature of the disease be understood.

The source of HSV inoculant for ocular herpes and herpetic whitlow (digital) is the saliva or direct contact with an active herpetic lesion. Extreme care must be taken to protect the eyes and any discontinuity of the skin (cuts, puncture wounds). Treatment for any form of herpetic lesion is still only palliative, to relieve pain and prevent secondary bacterial infection. (Refer to Chapter 3 for more details.)

Hepatitis

There are three viral agents that cause hepatitis: hepatitis A (HAV), hepatitis B (HBV), and non-A, non-B (NANB) sometimes known as HCV. The acute diseases caused by these agents are clinically indistinguishable, but they are virologically and immunologically different. Although approximately 60,000 cases of viral hepatitis are reported annually in the United States, this figure is thought to represent only a small percentage of actual cases. Estimates are that at least 100,000 cases of icteric HAV and at least 50,000 cases of icteric HBV occur each year, as well as several times this number of cases of anicteric HAV and HBV. Clinically, the outcome of acute hepatitis can range from asymptomatic to fulminant. In persons with HBV infection, approximately 6% to 10% of persons with acute HBV will become chronic carriers. According to James, about 13% of practicing general dentists contract HBV compared with 4% of the general population, while oral surgeons contract HBV six times more frequently than the general population. Feldman and Schiff found a significantly higher incidence of HBV in dentists than in lawyers in Dade County, Fla. (6.7% vs. 2.4%).

In addition, Mosley and coworkers noted that the more years of professional practice, the greater the likelihood of HBV infection. The HBV and perhaps NANB are of major concern to dental professionals.

Considering the inconvenience and potential cost of an acute illness requiring 4 to 6 weeks of absence from work, and considering the danger of becoming an HBV carrier, great concern over viral hepatitis as a hazard in dentistry is entirely appropriate. A new HBV vaccine is now commercially available to dentists and other high-risk people and has been reported to be highly effective. (See Smuzness and associates and *Morbidity and Mortality Weekly Report* 31:465-467, 1982.) It must be strongly emphasized, however, that stringent prophylactic measures described in Chapter 3 should still be taken to prevent hepatitis virus transmission.

AIDS

This is a relatively new and inadequately understood condition associated with an impairment in the body's immune system. Since 1978, a group of diseases associated with a specific defect in cell-mediated immunity has been recognized, manifested by Kaposi's sarcoma, *Pneumocystis carinii pneumonia* (PCP), *Toxoplasma gondii* infections, and other life-threatening opportunistic infections. This group of clinical entities is now called AIDS.

Persons that have been found to be primarily at risk are homosexual males, intravenous drug users, Haitians, and hemophiliacs. Although the number of reported cases to date exceeds 2,000, the true extent of the problem is not known. Symptoms include marked fatigue, persistent fevers or night sweats, weight loss unrelated to diet or activity, lymph node enlargement, discolored nodules on skin or mucous membranes, persistent dry cough, and diarrhea.

The etiology of the underlying immune deficiencies seen in AIDS cases is unknown. However, one hypothesis consistent with current observations is that a transmissible agent may be involved. The patterns of spread of the disease resemble the distribution and modes of spread of HBV, and infections with HBV occur very frequently among AIDS cases.

There is presently no evidence of AIDS transmission to hospital or dental personnel from contact with infected patients or clinical specimens. Nevertheless, because of concern about a possible transmissible agent, it would seem wise for such personnel to use the same precautions when caring for patients with AIDS as those used for patients with HBV infection, in which blood and body fluids likely to have been contaminated with blood are considered infective. Specifically, precautions should be taken to avoid direct contact of skin and mucous membranes with blood or blood products, excretions, secretions, and tissues of persons judged likely to have AIDS.

The importance of following recognized aseptic technique in the dental operatory cannot be overemphasized. Chapter 3 will be most useful in this regard.

Chemical Agents

Waste Anesthetic Gases

The administration of inhalation anesthesia in dental operatories has resulted in considerable exposure of dentists and their assistants to waste anesthetic agents. Although anesthetic gases have long been used in medicine and dentistry, their effects on the performance and well-being of those exposed and the reproductive effects from occupational exposure to the gases was not reported until 1967. Subsequent epidemiologic studies in the United States and in Europe have confirmed these findings, as have animal studies. Effects reported include decrements in motor, perceptual, and cognitive skills; liver disease; cancer; spontaneous abortions; and birth defects in offspring.

Perceptual, cognitive, and motor skills were studied by Bruce and associates in 40 male medical and dental students exposed on two occasions of 4 hours each by inhalation to either air or 500 ppm nitrous oxide with 5 ppm halothane. Compared with responses after breathing air, responses after exposure to nitrous oxide and halothane showed statistically significant decrements in the performance of tasks in which attention was divided between auditory and visual signals, a visual tachistoscopic test, and memory test involving digit span and recall of word pairs. After nitrous oxide alone, there were significant decrements in responses on digit test span only. Measurable decrements in performance of volunteers during testing at concentrations as low as 50 ppm nitrous oxide and 50 ppm nitrous oxide with 1 ppm halothane were noted in subsequent studies. Similar effects were not seen with 25 ppm nitrous oxide and 0.5 ppm halothane.

A study of dentists using inhalation anesthesia showed the spontaneous abortion rate to be increased by 78% ($P < .01$) in the wives of exposed dentists compared with the spouses of unexposed dentists. Congenital anomaly rates appeared to be slightly higher in the children of wives of exposed dentists than in the children of persons in the unexposed group, although the differences were not statistically significant.

NIOSH estimates that annually 100,000 dentists and dental assistants are exposed to waste anesthetic gases that include nitrous oxide, halothane, enflurane, and others. Studies by Whitcher and coworkers in dental operatories have indicated a mean concentration of 900 ppm of nitrous oxide in the breathing zone of the dentist, far in excess of the 50 ppm indicated by

NIOSH as achievable during analgesic dental anesthesia. Exposure to waste anesthetic gases occurs primarily from leakage of gases from the anesthetic system, poor fit of the masks on patients, and improper work practices including turning the equipment on before the patient is properly masked or not turning the system off before removing the mask. In addition, cleansing (blowing out) the system after use can release considerable residual gas from the tubing into the atmosphere, all of which contribute to staff exposure. (See Chapter 5 for more details.)

Airborne Particulates (Mineral Dusts)

Routine clinical dental procedures such as high-speed grinding of silica-containing composite restoratives, the contouring of fused porcelain, and the polishing of metals and plastics with silica or metallic oxides containing materials are not well characterized. However, the compositional and physical characteristics of some of the commonly employed dust-producing minerals closely resemble the features of minerals such as asbestos and silica that have been identified as causative agents in dust diseases of the lungs (pneumoconioses).

Asbestos has been used chiefly as a binder in periodontal dressings and as a lining material for casting rings and crucibles. Airborne asbestos has been known to cause pulmonary fibrosis (asbestosis), lung cancer, and mesothelioma of the pleura and peritoneum. Studies of airborne fibers of asbestos during preparation of gingivectomy packs have shown asbestos fibers in the atmosphere at inhalation levels 3 ft above the height of the table. The concern for the potential danger to dental personnel is sufficient that the Council on Dental Therapeutics no longer considers such products eligible for its acceptance program. Dentists should be aware of this occupational hazard and instead use packs that do not contain this material.

Methyl Methacrylate

The monomer component of methyl methacrylate is an irritant to the eyes, mucous membranes, and skin. Inhalation of the vapor causes salivation and conjunctival and respiratory irritation. Contact dermatitis can occur with skin contact. One study of pregnant rats exposed to methacrylate esters demonstrated embryofetal toxicity and teratogenic effects. Tansy and coworkers state that exposure of a human to methacrylate vapors results in a prompt decrease in gastric motor activity that lasts for 20 to 30 minutes after cessation of exposure. However, no data is available for prolonged exposure in humans or animals.

The necessary precautions for the use of this substance are described in Chapter 6.

Ethylene Oxide

The most common methods of sterilization in the dental office are auto-claving and submersion in a germicidal cleaner. These procedures offer minimal hazards, except for an occasional burn or dermatitis. However, ethylene oxide as a sterilant in dental offices is becoming more common. Excessive quantities of ethylene oxide (EtO) can be released from steriliz-ers during their routine use. NIOSH recommends that EtO in the work-place be regarded as a potential occupational carcinogen.

This recommendation is based on animal studies demonstrating EtO to be associated with increases in leukemia in female rats and peritoneal me-sotheliomas in male rats, evidence of mutagenicity in at least 13 biologic species, and limited epidemiologic investigations of two work sites suggest-ing an excess risk of cancer mortality among the EtO-exposed workers studied. In addition, EtO can cause skin, respiratory, and eye irritation; skin sensitization; nausea, vomiting, and diarrhea; and nervous system ef-fects. Male and female animal studies have demonstrated adverse effects on reproduction. Dental staff performing sterilization operations with EtO should be informed of its potential toxicity, and appropriate controls should be instituted to keep exposure to EtO as low as possible. Where control is not assured, alternate means for sterilization should be considered.

Mercury

Dental personnel are exposed to mercury toxicity through two primary sources: (1) contact or handling of mercury and mercury-containing com-pounds and (2) inhalation of vapors and respirable dusts.

The literature on mercury contamination in the dental office is vast. Ob-servations regarding safety range from reports of low risk to those of alarm-ing danger.

White and Brandt recently studied the development of mercury hyper-sensitivity among dental students. Members of the four 1972 to 1973 classes at the University of Texas Dental Branch at Houston and the incom-ing freshmen (a total of 396 volunteers) were patch-tested with a 0.1% aqueous solution of mercuric chloride and a 5% mixture of powdered silver amalgam in anhydrous lanolin.

The prefreshmen had no previous contact with amalgam at this point in their training, and all of the exposures to mercury involving the freshmen and most of the sophomores had resulted during training in restorative techniques. The results of this survey showed that there was a progressive increase in the development of hypersensitivity to mercury as students pro-gressed through dental school. The rates of mercury hypersensitivity, by class from prefreshmen to seniors, were 2.0%, 5.2%, 4.1%, 10.3%, and

10.8%, respectively. Twenty-two students displayed cutaneous reactions to the patches saturated with mercuric chloride, and five of these 22 displayed hypersensitivity to the patches with amalgam. No students had positive reactions to amalgam in the absence of a reaction to the mercuric chloride, and none were sensitive to lanolin alone. As a result of the continual contact with amalgam in dentistry, amalgam was considered to be the primary causative factor of the hypersensitivity. It was noted that the dental students in this study received only a small fraction of the exposure to mercury that a practicing dentist would receive, a fact that emphasizes the potential of the allergen in actual dental practice.

In order to investigate whether the babies of mothers occupationally exposed to low levels of elemental mercury had an increased mercury level, Wannay and Skjaerasen studied a group of 19 dentists, dental assistants, and dental technicians and compared them with a group of 26 nonexposed women. No measure of their workplace exposure to mercury was made, but it was inferred from other studies that the exposure was around the recommended threshold limit value of 0.05 mg/m^3 or lower. Tissue analyses indicated that the mercury content of the placenta in the exposed group (24.5 ng/g) was twice that of the unexposed (12 ng/g) and that both the chorion and amnion membrane showed corresponding difference between the exposed and the nonexposed group (21.6 ng/g and 11.5 ng/g for the chorion and 14.5 ng/g and 5.3 ng/g for the amnion membrane, respectively). The placentas of both groups and the chorion in the exposed group contained more mercury than the corresponding erythrocytes and plasma; the amount of mercury in the blood of mothers and babies in both groups at the time of delivery was similar. Concern for the effects of mercury on pregnancy is of particular importance with the increasing number of women dentists and the large number of women in the dental profession.

In a recent study by Ship and Shapiro, body mercury levels of a group of practicing dentists in the Delaware Valley were measured for both long-term and short-term accumulation. Those dentists with high mercury accumulation had neurologic and neuropsychological problems as well as deterioration in their visual graphic performance. Ship and Shapiro conclude that "the results of the study indicate that the current standards of mercury hygiene in dentistry are not consistent with safety in the dental office." This confirms Buchwald's study of mercury exposure to dental workers, where he notes that the most troublesome finding was the "general unawareness of the dentists, and especially their assistants, that mercury could be harmful, with the resulting almost total absence of even the most elementary precautionary measures."

Chapter 4 discusses these problems and provides the necessary information and resources to help control them.

Beryllium

Dental alloys may contain beryllium. Melting, grinding, buffing, and general lathing operations in the preparation of dentures can result in significant exposure to this highly toxic metal. Acute exposure to high concentrations of beryllium compounds can cause marked irritation of the eyes and respiratory tract, including the lung. Rom of the Rocky Mountain Center for Occupational and Environmental Health has recently reported three cases of acute chemical pneumonitis in dental laboratory technicians analagous to acute berylliousis as described by Denardi in the 1940s. The technicians had an overexposure from the grinding and melting of a non-precious alloy containing 2% beryllium. All three presented with dyspnea and reticulonodular infiltrates in their chest radiographs. Biopsies in these cases showed acute pneumonitis in one, interstitial changes with fibrosis in another, and granulomas in the third. In addition, Rom reports finding 2 of 7 personal samples for beryllium analysis taken on dental laboratory workers in Utah as being in excess of the OSHA permissible exposure limit of 2 μg/m^3 for 8 hours per day in a 40-hour week. Chronic exposure can produce delayed-onset pulmonary granulomatosis. Skin exposure has resulted in dermatitis, and beryllium metal or compounds implanted in lacerations may result in skin ulcers or granulomas.

Workrooms where operations involving beryllium are performed should be provided with effective ventilation to insure adequate control of this exposure, and care should be taken to protect the skin from such exposure.

Physical Agents

Ionizing Radiation

The benefits derived from the judicious use of radiography in modern dental practice are well known. It is important, however, that dental personnel understand the nature of radiation and its adverse effects and take the practical measures necessary to reduce the potential health hazards for themselves as well as for their patients.

Studies of radiologists in the 1940s and 1950s indicated a greater risk of leukemia and shorter life span for radiologists compared with other medical specialists. Warren has demonstrated that radiologists entering the field more recently have apparently taken greater precautions in regard to radiation protection and no longer stand out with statistically significant risk of shorter life span.

It is not clear, however, that dentistry is as fastidious with its precautions. This is likely due to less-than-adequate information about low-level ionizing radiation, which can lead to the careless and/or excessive use of x-rays. It is dismaying to note, for example, that a study done as late as 1969 of dentists in southwest England found that 38% of these dentists still held x-ray films in patients' mouths with some degree of regularity. Alcox remarks that dentists are "fond of defending their use of radiation . . . by telling (patients) that the dose that they receive is similar to that which they obtain from a day in the sun. . ."

This indicates that some dentists do not understand the difference between background radiation to the gonads and somatic doses of radiation in the oral cavity. Dental radiography does expose the head and neck areas of patients to radiation to a significant degree, and any exposure to ionizing radiation should be considered a potential hazard and be taken seriously. Since dentists or dental assistants take many more x-rays than are included in a single examination of the patient, the potential for their exposure is much greater for the dentists and dental staff if the x-ray operation is inadequately controlled. Smith claims that those dentists who are consistently careless and receive doses at the high end of the range (16 mR per month or 8 rad in the course of a working life) will have their annual chance of dying from leukemia increased by 20%. However, Warren and Lombard studied mortality rates of dentists in Massachusetts over a 6-year period (1959 to 1965) to determine whether radiation exposure contributed to an excess mortality ascribable to radiation use. They did not find such an excess and concluded that x-ray procedures now carried out are safe. In addition, Alcox notes that protection against radiation hazards has been improving as shown by the 1964 and 1970 x-ray exposure studies. Concern for radiation exposure, however, requires constant vigilance of the operating procedures and equipment. The individual practitioner might well take note of the information in Chapter 7 so that patient and worker exposure can be minimized in the dental office.

Ultraviolet and Visible Light Radiation

Dental personnel are exposed to ultraviolet radiation from several sources, such as devices for curing resins and sealants, plaque lights, and molten metal used in casting. Untoward effects of exposure include eye irritation, erythema of skin and/or mucous membranes, and malignant transformation of cells and viruses.

Visible light-cured resins, which are being used to a greater extent than those of ultraviolet curing, offer several advantages over the latter. However, there have been some reports, usually from animal studies, that state that retinal damage can occur as a result of continuous eye exposure. In either case, protective glasses and proper shielding are among the preventive measures discussed in Chapter 6.

Other Physical Agents

In addition to ionizing radiation, there are other physical agents that may have the potential to cause problems for the dental practitioner.

NOISE.—Noise, particularly that generated by the high-speed handpiece, is an occupational hazard that concerns dentists. Results of research on the subject are ambivalent. Taylor and coworkers examined 40 practicing dentists who had been exposed to the air-turbine drill for a median time of 3.7 years. They found that a 5- to 7-dB drop in hearing thresholds occurred at 4,000 and 6,000 Hz. Forman-Franco and associates, however, studied 70 dentists from eight specialities and found no significant decrease in hearing thresholds when compared with a normal age-adjusted population.

The American Conference of Governmental Industrial Hygienists (ACGIH) has adopted a slightly more stringent permissible 8-hour-day exposure limit for noise exposure than the 90-dB limit of OSHA. The ACGIH recommends that a maximum of a time-weighted average of 85 decibel-A scale (dBA) for a duration of 8 hours per day is permissible without causing damage, while 100 dBA is acceptable for 1-hour duration. The early ball-bearing dental handpiece at 12 in. measured 85 dBA, while the newer ball-bearing and air-bearing handpiece at 12 in. measures 75 dBA. The noise from these drills is not continuous for 8 hours, and the time-weighted average would be even lower. Technically, then, use of either type of drill should not cause permanent hearing impairment. Other variables must be considered, however, including intensity, age of handpiece, duration of exposure, distance to noise, and susceptibility of the operator.

ULTRASOUND.—There is currently no literature available about the potential hazard of ultrasound to the dental practitioner as a noise hazard.

Dermatitis

Contact dermatitis has been a problem among dentists for many years, at times incapacitating the practitioner and causing loss of productivity. The most common causes are soaps and detergents, because office personnel usually wash their hands well over 15 times each day. The most likely reason for these dermatoses is destruction of the protective layers of the epidermis. Consequently, hand cleaners should be used that do not contain abrasives, do not defat the skin, do not cause allergic sensitization, and do not break down with storage.

Other causes of dermatitis include direct contact with organic solvents and acids, which are predominantly used in bonding, etching, and fluoride treatments, as well as allergic reactions to certain substances such as epoxy resins and local anesthetics.

Preventive measures include avoiding contact with these irritating agents as much as possible and, where indicated, a sensitivity determination by a cutaneous patch test.

Chapter 6 covers the area of dermatitis more fully.

Musculoskeletal Disorders: Ergonomic Factors

Ergonomics is the study of the relationship between man, machines, and their environment. As applied to dentistry, the objective of such study is to reduce physical strain and mental fatigue of dental personnel and thereby increase their well-being and the quality and quantity of care given.

In 1974, Kajland and coworkers completed a study to determine the occupationally related medical problems of the dental profession. For the social and medical aspects of the study, they used interview and questionnaire techniques to survey 147 public health dentists and 92 controls (clerical workers matched by socioeconomic background). In addition, an ergonomic appraisal was made of these dentists (as well as 60 additional private-practice dentists) working under standardized conditions. This ergonomic evaluation was tested for covariation with reported musculoskeletal troubles. Disorders of the musculoskeletal system were reported to a significantly greater extent by dentists than by the control group. Also, a positive correlation was found between poor working positions and musculoskeletal problems. These findings were consistent with those of similar studies by others.

Factors to be evaluated include working positions (sitting and standing positions each have their own problems); lighting (including the relative intensities of operating and task-area lighting); noise levels and their effects on hearing; and equipment design, safety, and comfort (for both staff and patients). Chapter 9 should therefore be of considerable interest to the dental practitioner.

Injuries and Accidents

There are no complete statistics or case presentations indicating the actual number or severity of injuries that result in death or disability in the dental office. Although a great number probably occur daily, most are relatively minor, and there are no serious consequences. However, the seriousness of the situation should not be taken lightly. A survey of dentists by the ADA's Bureau of Economic Research and Statistics cited 17 cases of contusions, infections, or foreign objects in the eyes. Three practitioners lost eyes. It is important, therefore, that every dental professional be aware of the potential causes of accidents so that preventive measures may be taken (see Chapter 6).

Stress

A leading authority on stress research, Dr. Hans Selye, suggests that some stress is a necessary component of the experience of life. However, when stress becomes excessive to the point that it becomes harmful, Selye calls this "distress." When discussing stress, this negative connotation is implied.

The destructive aspects of stress are considered by some to be a greater threat to the dentist's health and well-being than any other ailment. Russek contends that results of clinical observation of coronary patients confirm the fact that "emotional stress of occupational origin may be far more significant in the etiologic picture of coronary disease than hereditary, dietary, fat, tobacco, obesity, or physical activity."

There are numerous factors that, alone or in combination, can cause stress in the modern dental practice, including physical confinement; dealing with patient anxiety; frustration in reaching treatment goals because of patient cost objections; high case loads; economic pressures; and interpersonal relationship problems, to name a few. Taking measures to reduce stress (as well as taking measures to improve the ability to cope with stress), therefore, is as important to the dentist's health as eliminating other occupational hazards. See Chapter 10 for more details.

REFERENCES

Acquired immune deficiency syndrome (AIDS): Precautions for clinical and laboratory staffs. *Morbidity Mortality Weekly Rep.* 31:43, 1982.

Alcox, Ray W.: Biological effects and radiation protection in the dental office. *Dent. Clin. North Am.* 22:517-533, 1979.

American Dental Association, Bureau of Economic and Behavioral Research: *Distribution of Dentists in the U.S. by State, Region, District and County.* Chicago, 1979.

American Dental Association, Bureau of Economic Research and Statistics: Mortality of dentists, 1951–1954. *J.A.D.A.* 52:65–72, 1956.

American Dental Association, Bureau of Economic Research and Statistics: Mortality of dentists, 1955–1960. *J.A.D.A.* 65:107–114, 1962.

American Dental Association, Bureau of Economic Research and Statistics: Mortality of dentists, 1961–1966. *J.A.D.A.* 76:831–834, 1968.

American Dental Association, Bureau of Economic Research and Statistics: Mortality of dentists, 1968–1972. *J.A.D.A.* 90:195–198, 1975.

American Dental Association, Bureau of Economic Research and Statistics: *The 1977 Survey of Dental Practice*. Chicago, 1978.

Autio K.L., Rosen S., Reynolds N.J., et al.: Studies on cross-contamination in the dental clinic. *J.A.D.A.* 100:358–361, 1980.

Brooks S.L., Rowe N.H., Drach J.C., et al.: Prevalence of herpes simples virus disease in a professional population. *J.A.D.A.* 102:31–34, 1981.

Bruce D.L., Bach M.J., Arbit J.: Trace anesthetic effects on perceptual, cognitive and motor skills. *Anesthesiology* 40:453–458, 1974.

Bruce D.L., Bach M.J.: *Trace Effects of Anesthetic Gases on Behavioral Performance of Operating Room Personnel*, publication 76-169. Cincinnati, U.S. Dept. of Health and Human Services, Public Health Service, National Institute for Occupational Safety and Health, 1976.

Buchwald H.: Exposure of dental workers to mercury. *Am. Indust. Hygiene Assoc. J.* 33:492–502, 1972.

Caruso R.J.: Dermatitis: A dentist's occupational hazard. *N.Y. State Dent. J.*, November 1981, pp. 543–545.

Cohen E.N., Brown B.W., Bruce D.L., et al.: A survey of anesthetic health hazards among dentists. *J.A.D.A.* 90:1291–1296, 1975.

Crawford J.J., cited by Committee Report of the North Carolina Dental Society: Suggested guidelines for asepsis in the dental office environment. *N.C. Dent. J.*, Winter-Spring, 1980.

Current Intelligence Bulletin 35: Ethylene Oxide, publication 81–130. U.S. Dept. of Health and Human Services, National Institute on Occupational Safety and Health, 1981.

Djerassi E.: Some problems of the occupational diseases of dentists. *Int. Dent. J.* 21:252–256, 1971.

Dyce J.M., Dow J.A.: Diagnosis and stress in dentistry. *Int. Dent. J.* 15:405, 1968.

Dyer M.R.: The possible adverse effects of asbestos in gingivectomy packs. *Br. Dent. J.* 122:507, 1967.

Feldman R.E., Schiff E.R.: Hepatitis in dental professionals. *J.A.M.A.* 232:1228–1230, 1975.

Forman-Franco B., Abramson A.L., Stein T.: High-speed drill noise and hearing: Audiometric survey of 70 dentists. *J.A.D.A.* 97:479–482, 1978.

Forrest W.R.: Stressed and self-destructive behavior of dentists. *Dent. Clin. North Am.* 22:367–371, 1978.

Francis D.P., Maynard J.E.: The transmission and outcome of hepatitis A, B and non-A and non-B: A review. *Epidemiol. Rev.* 1:17–31, 1979.

Glaser Z.R.: *Special Occupational Hazard Review with Control Recommendations for the Use of Ethylene Oxide as a Sterilant in Medical Facilities*, publication 77–200. U.S. Dept. of Health, Education and Welfare, National Institute on Occupational Safety and Health, 1977.

Hamilton A.: *Exploring the Dangerous Trades*. Boston, Little, Brown & Co., 1943.

Harley J.L.: Eye and facial injuries resulting from dental procedures. *Dent. Clin. North Am.* 22:505–515, 1978.

Harris N.D., Crabb L.J.: Ergonomics, reducing mental and physical fatigue in the dental operatory. *Dent. Clin. North Am.* 22:331–345, 1978.

Hepatitis B virus vaccine safety: Report of an interagency group. *Morbidity Mortality Weekly Rep.* 31(34):465–467, 1982.

Huget E.F., Cutright D.E.: Potential hazards in military dental practice. *Milit. Med.* 143:718–719, 1978.

James S., cited by Brown B.S.: Viral hepatitis B perspectives: Past and present. *Dent. Hygiene* 55:22–25, 1981.

Kajland A., Lindvall T., Nilsson T.: Occupational medical aspects of the dental profession. *Work Environ. Health* 11:100–107, 1974.

Katz C.: Reducing interpersonal stress in dental practice. *Dent. Clin. North Am.* 22:347–359, 1978.

Kuwabara, T., Gorn R.: Retinal damage by visible light. *Arch. Opthalmol.* 79:69, 1968.

La Rossa D., Hamilton R.: Herpes simplex infection of the digits. *Arch. Surg.* 102:600, 1971.

Mosley J.W., Edwards V.M., Casey G., et al.: Hepatitis B virus infection in dentists. *N. Engl. J. Med.* 293:729–734, 1975.

Muller S.A., Herrmann E.C.: Association of stomatitis and paronychias due to herpes simplex. *Arch. Dermatol.* 101: 396, 1970.

NIOSH Criteria for a Recommended Standard. . . .Occupational Exposure to Waste Anesthetic Gases and Vapor, publication 77–140. U.S. Dept. of Health, Education and Welfare, National Institute on Occupational Safety and Health, 1977.

Nystrom A., cited by Kajland A., Lindvall T., Nilsson T.: Occupational medical aspects of the dental profession. *Work Environ. Health* 11:100–107, 1974.

Occupational Mortality, 1921. The Registrar General's Decennial Supplement, England and Wales, 1927. London, Her Majesty's Stationery Office, 1927.

Occupational Mortality, 1931. The Registrar General's Decennial Supplement, England and Wales, 1927. London, Her Majesty's Stationery Office, 1938.

Occupational Mortality, 1951. The Registrar General's Decennial Supplement, England and Wales, 1927. London, Her Majesty's Stationery Office, 1958.

Occupational Mortality, 1961. The Registrar General's Decennial Supplement, England and Wales, 1927. London, Her Majesty's Stationery Office, 1971.

Orner G., Breslin P.: *Mortality Study of Dentists,* Contract No. HSM99–72–72. U.S. Department of Health, Education and Welfare, 1976.

Park P.R.: Effects of sound on dentists. *Dent. Clin. North Am.* 22:415–429, 1978.

Part of the Human Condition, Publication 78–137. U.S. Dept. of Health and Human Services, National Institute for Occupational Safety and Health, 1978.

Potts P.: Chirurgical Observations Relative to the Cataract, the Polypus of the Nose, the Cancer of the Scrotum, the Different Kind of Ruptures and the Mortification of the Toes and Feet, London, 1775, cited by Hunter D: *The Diseases of Occupation,* ed. 5. London, English Universities Press, 1975.

Proctor N.H., Hughes J.P.: *Chemical Hazards of the Workplace.* Philadelphia, J.B. Lippincott, Co., 1978.

Ramazzini B.: *De Morbis Artificium Diatriba,* Geneva, 1713, Wright W.C. (trans.-ed.). Chicago, University of Chicago Press, 1940.

Reports of Councils and Bureaus: Hazards of asbestos in dentistry. *J.A.D.A.* 92:777–778, 1976.

Rom W.: Personal communication, Salt Lake City, Utah, 1983–1984.

Russek H.I.: Emotional stress and coronary heart disease in American physicians, dentists and lawyers. *Am. J. Med. Sci.* 243:716–725, 1962.

Sand M.A., Gadot F., Wenzel R.P.: Point source epidemic of Mycoplasmic pneumoniae infection in a prosthodontics laboratory. *Am. Rev. Respir. Dis.* 112:213–217, 1975.

Schafer W.G., Hine M.K., Levy B.M.: *A Textbook of Oral Pathology.* Philadelphia, W.B. Saunders Co., 1974.

Ship I.I., Shapiro I.M.: Preventing mercury poisoning in dental practice. *Compendium of Continuing Education on General Dentistry,* March 1, 1983.

Singh A.R., Lawrence W.H., Autian J.: Embryonic-fetal toxicity and teratogenic effects of a group of methacrylate esters in rats. *Appl. Pharmacol.* 22:314–315, 1972.

Smith N.J.D.: The hazard to the dentist and his staff from dental radiology. *Dent. Practitioner Dent. Record* 27:409–413, 1972.

Smuzness W.E., Stevens C.E., Harley E.J., et al.: Hepatitis B vaccine: Demonstration of efficacy in a controlled clinical trial in high-risk population in the United States. *N. Engl. J. Med.* 303:833–841, 1980.

Tansy M.F., Benhoyem S., Probst S., et al.: The effects of methyl methacrylate vapor on gastric motor function. *J.A.D.A.* 89:372–376, 1974.

Taylor W., Pearson J., Mair A.: The hearing threshold levels of dental practitioners exposed to air turbine drill noise. *Br. Dent. J.* 118:206, 1965.

Travaglini E.A., Larato D.C., Martin A.: Dissemination of organism-bearing droplets by high-speed dental drills. *J. Prosthet. Dent.* 16:132–139, 1966.

Ulrich H.: The incidence of leukemia in radiologists. *N. Engl. J. Med.* 234:45–46, 1946.

Vaisman A.I., cited by Cohen E.N., Brown B.W., Bruce D.L., et al.: A survey of anesthetic health hazards among dentists. *J.A.D.A.* 90:1291–1296, 1975.

Wannay A., Skjaerasen J.: Mercury accumulation in placenta and foetal membranes: A study of dental workers and their babies. *Environ. Phys. Biochem.* 5:348–352, 1975.

Warren S.: Longevity and causes of death from irradiation in physicians. *J.A.M.A.* 162:464, 1956.

Warren S.: The basis for the limit on whole-body exposure-experience of radiologists. *Health Phys.* 12:737, 1966.

Warren S., Lombard O.M.: Mortality and radiation exposure of Massachusetts dentists. *J.A.D.A.* 80:329–330, 1979.

Whitcher C.E., Zimmerman D.C., Piziali R.L.: *Control of Occupational Exposure to N_2O in the Dental Operatory,* publication 77–171. U.S. Dept. of Health, Education and Welfare, National Institute on Occupational Safety and Health, 1977.

White R.R., Brandt R.L.: Development of mercury hypersensitivity among dental students. *J.A.D.A.* 92:1204–1207, 1976.

Chapter 2

Aerosol Hazards*

Robert L. Cooley, D.M.D., M.S.

DENTAL AEROSOLS may be defined as suspensions of extremely fine airborne particles that are liquid, solid, or combinations of both. Aerosol particles are microscopic and are generally described as being less than 50 μ in diameter, which allows them to remain suspended in air for long periods of time. The definition of an aerosol implies that the suspension may persist for over 24 hours. The particles may settle out of suspension over a period of time, but also may be carried considerable distances from their origin before this "settling out" occurs.

The major hazard arising from aerosols is associated with their small particle size, which allows them to enter the respiratory system. Particle size in dental aerosols has been shown to vary greatly, ranging from 50 μ to less than 0.5 μ. The degree to which they penetrate the respiratory system is dependent on the aerodynamic diameter of the particle. The aerodynamic diameter of a particle is equivalent to the diameter of a spherical particle of unit density, having the same settling velocity in air. The larger the aerodynamic diameter, the higher in the respiratory system it is deposited. The particles with smaller aerodynamic diameters can penetrate to the lungs and be deposited in the alveoli. Deposition of the particles will generally occur in the following manner:

Aerodynamic Diameter	Respiratory Penetration
0.5 – 5 μ	Lungs < Alveoli / Bronchioles
5 – 10 μ	Nasal pharynx, pharynx, trachea
10 – 50 μ	Nose and upper airways

There may be some overlap in the deposition of various size particles within the respiratory system. The deposition site may be altered by the effect of humidity on water-soluble particles, which can increase their size, or also by an electrical charge on particles that are less than 0.1 μ.

---

*The views and opinions expressed herein are those of the author and do not necessarily reflect the views of the United States Air Force or the Department of Defense.

Aerosol Particle Characteristics

* 50 μ diameter is maximum particle size in aerosols.
* 95% of particles have diameter of less than 5 μ.
* Particles remain airborne for over 24 hours.
* 75% of particles are contaminated with microorganisms.
* 95% can reach the alveoli of the lungs.
* Particles can travel on air currents to other rooms.

Hazard to Dental Personnel

Air-turbine handpieces, air-water sprays, some rotary instruments, ultrasonic scalers, and dental lathes all produce aerosols that have the potential for causing disease due primarily to inhalation. There are a number of studies that demonstrate the production of aerosols from various instruments, as well as the composition and extent of the aerosol. Dental aerosols may have three components that should be of particular interest to the dentist and his staff:

* Bacteria and viruses
* Particles of tooth structure
* Particles of dental materials

Bacteria and Viruses In Aerosols

Bacteria and viruses can become components of dental aerosols during many types of procedures. Most investigators of aerosols have expressed a concern that these organisms can enter the respiratory system or the eye and produce disease. The disease processes most often cited include the following:

Disease	Source
Herpetic lesions of the eye	Virus from herpetic oral and lip lesions
Tuberculosis	Tubercle bacilli from open lesions
Influenza or common cold	Virus from infected patients
Conjunctivitis	Various organisms such as staphylococcus

Micik and associates have performed a number of aerosol studies that have compared the number of bacteria produced by dental procedures with that produced by coughing and sneezing. In a controlled environment operatory, they found the following three procedures to produce bacteria in numbers similar to coughing: (1) prophylaxis procedure using a pumice cup and pumice, (2) air-turbine handpiece with air coolant, and (3) air spray from an air-water syringe. However, the use of air-water spray with the air-turbine handpiece increased the airborne bacteria 20 times and was comparable to sneezing in ability to atomize bacteria. Bristle brushes and the air-water spray from a three-way syringe produced greater bacterial aerosols than coughing or sneezing. These same studies demonstrated that a high-velocity suction would reduce the bacterial aerosol by 96% to 99%.

Larato and coworkers also studied bacterial aerosols produced by the air-turbine handpiece and found that during cavity preparations, the airborne bacteria increased 2,200%. Other investigators have noted that high bacterial counts were generated when the air turbine was used in any quadrant of the mouth. Working at distances of 15 to 20 in. from the mouth, there appeared to be no zone of safety from this bacterial-contaminated mist.

Particulate Aerosols of Tooth Structure and Dental Materials

Several investigators have demonstrated that aerosols of enamel, dentin, amalgam, and composite resin are produced during high-speed cutting or finishing. Of particular interest is a study by Madden and associates, who evaluated the effect of water-flow rates and bur shapes on aerosol particle size. It was found that 99% of these aerosols contained particles of 5 μ or less. These investigators indicated that 95% of the particles in the aerosol could travel to the alveoli of the lung and possibly represent a serious health hazard. They also discovered that the water-flow rate through the air-turbine handpiece had a considerable effect on the aerosol production. The greater the flow rate, the greater the amount of aerosol generated that was also rich in the smaller particles.

Timbrell and Eccles investigated the respirability of aerosols produced by both clinical and laboratory procedures. They found that the water spray would not prevent aerosols of enamel and dentin particles. The water spray did show some ability in limiting the number of particles, but did not eliminate particles of tooth debris in the aerosol. When enamel and dentin were cut with an air turbine without a water spray, a fine aerosol was produced that had a large portion of particles that could reach the alveolar regions of the lung. The use of a high-velocity suction was recommended to reduce the aerosol and lower the health risk.

Concern has also been expressed over the fact that these particles of tooth debris and dental materials are contaminated with microorganisms. Several studies have indicated that 75% of these minute particles are contaminated. Some believe that these particles and droplets of water may serve as vehicles to transport the microbes into the lungs.

One dental material in particular, alginate, has been singled out for several studies to determine its contribution to dental aerosols. Silicon has been shown to be the chief inorganic constituent of alginate. Evaluation of airborne alginate particles reveals that 10% to 15% are silicon fibers. Alginate dust can be seen rising from containers that have been tumbled to mix the powder and also from vigorous spatulation during mixing. Two investigations of the alginate aerosol concluded that overexposure is not likely to occur during spatulation or opening of the container. However, others have noted that the alginate aerosol contains fibers, 10% to 15% of which are similar to asbestos fibers that are known to cause lung malignancies in asbestos workers. These fibers are 20 μ in length and 3 μ in diameter, which is in the size range considered to present the highest risk. Concern has been expressed that these fibers may collect in the lung over a long period of time and have a cumulative effect that could possibly result in fibrosis or carcinoma. However, as yet, there do not appear to be any proven cases of lung disease as a result of inhalation of alginate aerosols.

Dental Personnel at Risk

1. Dentist
2. Dental assistant
3. Hygienist
4. Laboratory technician
5. Additional office personnel

Dentists, dental assistants, and hygienists are exposed to aerosols that may contain bacteria, viruses, tooth debris, or particles of dental materials and should be considered at risk. Patients exposed to these contaminated mists may be at some risk of cross contamination from other patients because of the long period of time these minute particles can remain suspended in air. Laboratory technicians may be exposed to bacterial aerosols when polishing dentures or appliances that have been in the mouth. In addition, many of their procedures involve the grinding or polishing of various dental materials that could create an aerosol. As for other personnel, such as receptionists or clerks, there is some indication that they may be exposed to aerosols created in the laboratory or operatory. It has been demonstrated that bacterial aerosols created by polishing dentures with contaminated pumice can be distributed throughout a dental office by a forced-air heating/cooling system. Perhaps even more indicative of the risk was the discovery that these same bacteria could be detected in the nose and pharynx of patients in the other rooms of the dental office. Therefore, it appears that these aerosols have the ability to travel on air currents and contaminate individuals in all areas of the dental office, and not just those at the source of the aerosol.

Sources of Aerosol

Table 2–1 lists various aerosol sources. Any of the instruments listed can produce a bacterial aerosol in the presence of bacterial plaque, normal oral flora, or an active disease. The water spray from an air-turbine handpiece has been demonstrated to produce a bacterial aerosol when operated in the mouth, even though *not* actually cutting tooth structure. The air-water spray may produce aerosols with 20 times more bacteria than when the water is turned off and air used alone. In addition, the air-water spray from a three-way syringe has been shown to propel bacteria from the mouth in numbers greater than coughing or sneezing. Ultrasonic scalers may increase the airborne bacterial concentration by 3,000%.

Pumice containers for dental lathes become quickly contaminated when dentures or appliances directly from the mouth are polished. When con-

TABLE 2–1.—SOURCES OF AEROSOL

BACTERIAL-VIRAL

Oral
Normal oral flora
Bacterial plaque
Calculus
Respiratory disease
Herpetic lesions
Pulmonary tuberculosis
Caries
Intraoral infections

Extraoral
Contaminated pumice from dental lathes
Contaminated water supply from dental units

PARTICULATES

Enamel
Dentin
Amalgam
Composite resins
Porcelain
Acrylics
Various metals
Alginates

INSTRUMENTS PRODUCING AEROSOLS

Air-turbine handpiece
Air-water syringe
Ultrasonic scalers
Rotary brushes and wheels
Rag wheels and brushes on dental lathes
Prophylaxis cups
Air-abrasive
   prophylaxis instruments

taminated pumice or rag wheels are used for polishing, the bacteria or virus can be atomized and eventually carried to all areas of the dental office by air currents.

Tests on the water from dental units indicate that the water lines may become contaminated with bacteria. Miller and Micik have described this bacterial contamination as massive when compared with city-supplied chlorinated water. These microorganisms are believed to enter the water lines through the handpieces or water syringes and may actually be siphoned or aspirated into the water lines by a back-siphonage phenomena. The water spray from these instruments could produce a bacterial aerosol to which the dentist, assistant, and patient will be exposed.

Role of Aerosols in Disease

The relationship between aerosols and disease has not been completely defined. There have been a number of investigations concerning the effect of aerosols on dental personnel and laboratory technicians, but there is still some controversy on this subject. Studies in the late 1930s and early 1940s found that laboratory technicians who performed grinding and polishing procedures had a high percentage of silicosis. Other investigations found that the death rate from respiratory diseases among dentists doubled from 1960 to 1972, which some have attributed to the aerosols generated by air-turbine handpieces. Several other studies have implied that there was a direct relationship between the use of the air-turbine handpiece and respiratory illness. Two studies of dental students also support the causal relationship between aerosols and respiratory disease. In the first, dental students were found to have a consistently higher incidence of respiratory disease than either medical or pharmacy students. In the second, there was a dramatic increase in positive tuberculin tests between junior and senior dental students. This increase was from 5% positive at the beginning of the junior year to 33% positive by the end of the senior year.

However, not all studies have demonstrated that dental aerosols pose a high risk to health. The results of an investigation on Navy dentists and their patients indicated that aerosols posed only a low-to-moderate risk of infection, and these investigators concluded that the airborne route of infection is not as great a hazard as has been speculated.

The question of whether a patient is at risk when exposed to dental aerosols has not been completely answered either. From what is currently known, there does not appear to be a direct relationship between certain respiratory diseases and dental aerosols.

Clinical Detection of Aerosols

Methods of detecting and sampling aerosols are available, but are not required. However, it has been clearly established that these contaminated mists are present when certain instruments are used. Therefore, one's efforts should be directed at eliminating or reducing this potential hazard to health.

Preventive Measures

There are many procedures and devices that will either minimize the production of aerosols or prevent them from being inspired:

Most Commonly Recommended Items

- Face masks and safety glasses
- Rubber dam
- Suction (high velocity)
- Preoperative mouthrinse
- Good ventilation
- Avoid patients with respiratory infections

Other Recommendations

- Avoid use of bristle wheels.
- Prevent pumice contamination.
- Sterilize rag wheels for dental lathe.
- Use suction for dental lathe.
- Use suction for all laboratory grinding procedures.
- Prohibit smoking.
- Spray operatory with disinfectant.
- Wipe all surfaces with disinfectant.
- Flush water lines on dental unit.
- Use high-efficiency particulate air (HEPA) or electrostatic filters.
- Use laminar airflow.

FACE MASKS AND SAFETY GLASSES.—These are probably the most recommended items for protection against aerosols. Safety glasses will protect the eyes from droplets containing bacteria and viruses as well as particles of tooth and amalgam that may be contaminated with microorganisms. A well-fitted, efficient face mask can greatly reduce the bacteria or particulate matter being inspired by the dentist, assistant, or laboratory technician.

Obviously, a mask that does not fit well, allowing leaks around the edges, will not provide adequate filtration. Selecting an efficient mask may not be easy, but several manufacturers now claim efficiency rates of between 96% and 99%. One recent study on dust in dental laboratories found mask efficiency rates of 70% to 95%, although smaller particles of less than 5 μ were not filtered. Some masks have proven to be 99% effective in bacterial filtration. Rogers' evaluation of the efficiency of disposable face masks found that many surgical masks protect the patient better than the wearer. However, several of the surgical masks performed well and were very effective at filtering out microorganisms to protect the wearer. The more effective masks are listed below:

Mask	Efficiency For Wearer (%)
Deseret E-Z Breathe	98–99
Deseret (no glass)	94–97
3M 1818	98–99
Bard International	96–98
Bard Vigilon	98–99
Surgine	99

Molded composition and paper masks in general were judged inefficient in this study and did not provide good protection for the wearer. An efficient, well-fitting face mask is highly recommended, because it will significantly reduce the bacterial and particulate matter being inspired.

RUBBER DAM.—The use of a rubber dam isolates much of the oral flora and bacterial plaque from the atomizing action of the air-turbine handpiece and air-water syringe. In some cases, it may prevent blood from being atomized or ejected from the mouth as droplets. The use of a rubber dam is highly recommended whenever possible.

HIGH-VELOCITY SUCTION.—The use of a high-velocity suction has been shown to be extremely effective at reducing aerosol concentrations. Some investigators have found that effective use of suction will reduce the aerosol concentration by 1,000 times. The use of this device is highly recommended for all procedures.

PREOPERATIVE MOUTHRINSE.—The use of a bactericidal mouthwash can significantly reduce the oral flora and the number of microorganisms in dental aerosols. Mouthwashes have been shown to reduce oral flora by 76% to 96% and the number of bacteria in aerosols by 89%. One mouthwash with a quaternary ammonium compound component was found to be more effective than tooth brushing in reducing the numbers of bacteria in aerosols. The use of this procedure is highly recommended.

GOOD VENTILATION.—Good ventilation is the key to the removal and clearance of airborne microorganisms from the dental treatment room. It is probably the single most important item that can be utilized to reduce the various air contaminants such as bacterial and particulate aerosols, mercury vapors, nitrous oxide, and various chemical vapors. An adequate airflow will dilute all these contaminants as well as aid in their removal. It has been demonstrated that as few as two room-air exchanges per hour will remove 90% of the airborne particles. However, some authorities such as the Centers for Disease Control recommend a minimum of six air exchanges per hour. The ventilation system of a dental facility should receive considerable attention during new construction or remodeling with the goal of making it as effective as funds and technology permit. If adequate ventilation is not possible, the use of an electrostatic or high-efficiency particulate air filter should be considered and will be discussed later in this section.

AVOID PATIENTS WITH RESPIRATORY INFECTIONS.—Common sense dictates that one should not perform elective treatment on patients with respiratory infections. The same microorganisms that are causing the patient's illness can be atomized and inspired by the dental staff as well as contaminate the office and instruments.

AVOID BRISTLE WHEELS AND BRUSHES.—Some bristle wheels and brushes utilized in polishing amalgam restorations have been shown to significantly increase the numbers of bacteria in aerosols. The aerosols created by bristle wheels exceed those produced by coughing and sneezing. It has been recommended that finishing burs and rubber points be substituted for these rotary instruments because they atomize far less microorganisms.

REDUCING AEROSOLS FROM DENTAL LATHES.—Pumice can quickly become contaminated when dentures or appliances are removed directly from the mouth and polished. Each time this contaminated pumice is used, bacterial aerosols are created. To avoid this problem, it has been suggested that a small amount of fresh pumice be used for each procedure and then discarded. The rag wheels and brushes should be sterilized each time that they are used on a denture or appliance that has been in the mouth. This sterilization may be accomplished with either an autoclave or a chemiclave. The rag wheel can be stored in a sterilization bag until needed. This contamination may also be reduced by scrubbing the appliance or denture with a disinfectant such as iodine-based compounds. In addition, the dental lathe should be operated in conjunction with a suction. One type of vacuum system for the dental lathe demonstrated a 3,000-fold reduction in aerosols. Units containing both a dental lathe and built-in suction are commercially available.

USE SUCTION FOR ALL LABORATORY GRINDING PROCEDURES.—A good suction system should be provided for all laboratory procedures where grinding of dental materials occur. These suction systems have been shown to effectively control dust from grinding of dental materials. Without good ventilation or suction, the particulate level of various dental materials may exceed the safe level. Studies of dental laboratories with poor or improper ventilation identified dust levels of several materials that exceeded the safe level or TLV (threshold limit value). Levels of mercury, silver, cobalt, and gypsum were 10 times the safe level, and in one situation, the silver level was 1,750 times the safe level.

PROHIBIT SMOKING.—Smoking should not be allowed in the dental office because tobacco smoke may interfere with some types of air-clearance systems and is for well-known reasons considered an unhealthy practice.

SPRAY OPERATORY WITH DISINFECTANT.—Recommendations for reducing bacterial aerosols have included spraying the operatory with disinfectants. Propylene glycol and triethylene glycol may be somewhat effective at killing staphylococci and influenza viruses; however, the glycol sprays have been shown to be no more effective than a water spray in reducing the number of airborne bacteria. From the more recent studies, one can conclude that aerosol disinfectant sprays have either limited or no effectiveness in reducing airborne microorganisms and the risk of infection from this source. Good ventilation appears to be the key in reducing bacterial/viral aerosols. If it is not possible to obtain proper ventilation or if a disinfectant spray is desired, then it should be applied to the treatment room at the end of the work day. Some of these agents may have an objectionable odor or be irritating, and the effects of breathing the disinfectant over a long period of time are not known.

WIPE ALL SURFACES WITH DISINFECTANT.—Cabinets and counters can become contaminated from dental aerosols. While this contamination probably does not contribute significantly to bacterial aerosols, it is included here to present an improved method of decontamination. Sodium hypochlorite (or laundry bleach) can be diluted to form a very effective germicidal solution. A 1% solution or 50:1 dilution is reported to be very effective against vegetative bacteria and may also prove effective against other organisms such as the hepatitis B virus. Another acceptable disinfecting solution can be made by mixing alcohol with an iodine compound (such as Betadine®). One suggested ratio is 20 parts of isopropyl alcohol with one part Betadine, which has 1% active iodine. Gloves should be worn and some care observed with the use of this solution, because the iodine component may stain some materials and fabrics as well as cause corrosion of some metals. The alkaline glutaraldehydes have also been shown to be very effective for disinfection. The glutaraldehydes may cause irritation of the skin and eyes; therefore, rubber gloves or forceps should be employed to prevent skin contact.

FLUSH WATER LINES ON DENTAL UNITS.—Water from dental units has been shown to be contaminated with bacteria. This problem may be particularly obvious on a Monday morning when the unit is first turned on and there is a musty or moldy odor to the water spray. The bacteria may enter the water lines through the handpieces by being aspirated into the water lines through a back-siphonage or back-flow of the water each time it is turned off. Flushing of the water lines each morning to remove the contaminated water is highly recommended. Studies of this problem have shown that a 1-minute flush can reduce the bacterial concentration by up to 97%, and a 2-minute flush can provide a 98.6% reduction. When flushing is accomplished, the handpieces should be disconnected from the air-water lines to allow drainage and thus prevent the aerosolization of this contaminated water. Miller and Micik developed an auxiliary pressurized water tank to supply chlorinated water to the dental unit, which greatly reduced the bacterial contamination of the water lines. Commercial water units are now available that supply sterile water to the dental unit, and methods to provide periodic chemical disinfection of unit water lines are being investigated. Antiretraction valves that prevent this back-siphonage or back-flow of water and hopefully prevent bacterial contamination are also available for dental units. A dental unit can be checked for this aspiration or back-siphonage of water by running the air-turbine handpiece in a cup of red disclosing solution. The handpiece is then disconnected and the handpiece controller activated. If any of the red dye comes out of the water lines or if any red dye is discovered in the lines of the handpiece, back-flow is occurring.

USE HEPA OR ELECTROSTATIC FILTERS.—Use of HEPA filters or electrostatic filters has been shown to be effective in reducing the airborne concentration of microorganisms. One study of these units indicated that they can reduce the microbial concentration by 50% for every 5 minutes of operation. If the practitioner has an operatory with poor ventilation, he may want to consider the use of one of these devices. They are available as floor or portable models and are sold by various retailers. Electrostatic filters installed within the ventilation system of dental laboratories have demonstrated a reduction of gypsum dust by 98% and gold dust by 60%. However, these filter systems should not be substituted for a high-velocity suction system in either the operatory or laboratory, because the suction system is very effective in preventing the aerosol at its origin. The high-velocity suction system has been shown to reduce the aerosol concentration in the operatory by 1,000 times.

USE LAMINAR AIRFLOW.—The laminar airflow system is one that circulates all the air in the operatory along parallel lines at a constant speed. This is accomplished with an electric blower that moves the air from the ceiling to the floor and then recirculates it through a HEPA filter. These systems have been found to be extremely effective at reducing the airborne microbial concentration (by as much as 97%). These systems would be expensive to install in an existing office, but could be easily designed into a new facility.

Splatter

Although splatter is not an aerosol, some mention and recognition should be made of those larger particles that are projected out of the mouth. Splatter is a term used by Micik and coworkers to describe airborne particles composed of water, bacteria, and other particulate matter. This is the material that can be seen on spectacles or safety glasses after the use of the air-turbine handpiece. It may also be projected onto counter tops, cabinets, chairs, dental units, and onto the dentist and assistant. These airborne particles can enter the eye, nose, mouth, or contact the lips. Splatter can carry significant numbers of bacteria and has been equated to bacterial aerosols for degree of contamination. Splatter presents a different problem than aerosols in that its microbial concentration is not reduced by the use of a suction, rubber dam, or preoperative mouthwash. Some protective measures have been suggested as follows:

- Use face mask and safety glasses.
- Avoid instruments that produce splatter (bristle wheels).
- Reduce water pressure of air-water syringe to prevent bounce-back effect of the water.
- Avoid use of water-spray combination: use water separately followed by air.

REFERENCES

Larato D., Ruskin P., Martin A., et al.:Effect of a dental air turbine drill on the bacterial counts in air. *J. Prosthet. Dent.* 16:758, 1966.

Legan J.L., Madden R., Thoma B., et al.: Biologic exposure to dental materials. *Oral Surg.* 36:908, 1973.

Lu D.P., Zambito R.F.: Aerosols and cross infection in dental practice: A historic view. *Gen. Dent.* 29, 1981.

Madden R.M., Hausler W., Leaverton P.: Study of some factors contributing to aerosol production by the air turbine handpiece. *J. Dent. Res.* 48:341, 1969.

Micik R.E., Miller R.L., Mazzarella M.A., et al.: Studies on dental aerobiology: I. Bacterial aerosols generated during dental procedures. *J. Dent. Res.* 48:49, 1969.

Miller R.L., Micik R.E.: Air pollution and its control in the dental office. *Dent. Clin. North Am.* 22:453, 1978.

Occupational Diseases: A Guide To Their Recognition. National Institute For Occupational Safety and Health, U.S. Government Printing Office, June 1977.

Rogers K.B.: An investigation into the efficiency of disposable face masks. *J. Clin. Pathol.* 33:1086, 1980.

Shreve W.B., Tow H.D.: Bacteriological and serological surveillance of dentists exposed to dental aerosols. *Bull. Tokyo Med. Dent. Univ.* 22:151, 1981.

Timbrell V., Eccles J.D.: The respirability of aerosols produced in dentistry. *J. Dent.* 12:21, 1973.

Chapter 3

Infectious and Communicable Diseases*

Kenton S. Hartman, D.D.S., M.S.D.

FRICK ESTIMATES that as many as 45% of all dentists believe they have contracted infectious illnesses in professional practice. The chances for dental personnel to contract a variety of infectious diseases can be appreciated when one considers that 1 in every 5 patients is a carrier of *Staphylococcus aureus*, 1 in every 10 is a carrier of *Streptococcus pyogenes*, 1 in every 200 may be a carrier of hepatitis B, and so on. Dentists in private practice may average 3,500 or more patient visits per year. This frequency of exposure to the microbial flora of the oral cavity through contaminated blood, saliva, aerosols, and splatter increases the likelihood of exposure to pathogenic microorganisms among dentists, dental assistants, dental hygienists, and laboratory personnel. Upper respiratory tract infections, especially colds and flu, are overall the most commonly contracted illnesses, and the potential for infection increases during the winter and spring seasons. According to the Fauchard Academy poll, hand and finger infections have been reported in 14% of dental practitioners, and another 9% have been afflicted with eye infections.

There are only a few epidemiologic studies to date that correlate the rate of microbial infection between dental personnel and the general public. There is no doubt that dental personnel are at increased risk of acquiring hepatitis B, herpetic or syphilitic paronychias, tuberculosis, and several other dieseases in comparison with the general public, but well-controlled epidemiologic studies to assess the overall importance of these diseases to dental professionals are incomplete.

Bacteria, viruses, and fungi represent the most common groups of microorganisms confronting dental professionals as infectious disease hazards. The capability of these organisms to produce disease requires a portal of entry into the body and a susceptible host. Primary exposure areas in den-

---

*The views and opinions expressed herein are those of the author and do not necessarily reflect the views of the United States Air Force or the Department of Defense.

tistry are skin, respiratory, and mucous membrane surfaces of the mouth, nasopharynx, and eyes. Natural barriers to infection are present at these portals of entry. When intact, the skin integument is a very effective covering that is impervious to most infectious agents, and the fatty acids in its secretions can inhibit growth of some microorganisms. The respiratory tract is coated with mucous and has a complex system of cilia along with a cough reflex to entrap and expel microorganisms. Tears and saliva contain substances such as lysozymes and proteolytic enzymes that can inhibit the growth of many microorganisms. Once these initial defense systems are penetrated and the invading microbes have gained access into the tissues, they are then confronted with the destructive power of the body's immune system and the inflammatory process. We all possess a very capable natural defense system in combating infectious diseases; however, it behooves us not to accept additional or unnecessary risks in dental practice by not following common sense measures for infection control.

Bacterial Infections

Dental personnel are routinely exposed to a wide variety of bacterial organisms that may cause skin, eye, and respiratory infections. Any of these allegedly "minor" infections are capable of causing an incapacitating condition resulting in loss of productive time in a dental practice. Although intact skin is remarkably resistant to infections, small breaks in the skin caused by minor cuts or abrasions allow for invasion of the skin by microorganisms. In both temperate and tropical climates, the great majority of bacterial skin infections are caused by two species of gram-positive cocci: S. pyogenes (β-hemolytic streptococci, group A) and S. aureus (coagulase-positive staphylococci).

Impetigo

Streptococci are believed to be incapable of invading intact skin and therefore require a portal of entry to create an infection. Streptococcal infections differ from staphylococcal infections in regard to spread of infection through the tissues; streptococcal infections tend to spread rapidly via the lymphatics, resulting in ascending lymphangitis. Streptococci cause a variety of cutaneous infections including impetigo, cellulitis, erysipelas, and fasciitis. Cutaneous streptococcal infections other than erysipelas are referred to collectively as streptococcal pyoderma. The lesions of streptococcal impetigo occur mainly on the extremities and do not commonly affect the face and head as does staphylococcal impetigo (bullous impetigo). Bullous impetigo is a superficial staphylococcal skin infection that involves the face and head, particularly around the nose and mouth. The disease principally affects infants and children and develops into thin-walled vesicles that quickly rupture, leaving dried, honey-colored crusts that adhere to the skin. These patients are not highly contagious to dental personnel, but routine precautions such as the wearing of rubber gloves are indicated. Treatment of bullous impetigo is essentially rupture of the bullae with local hygiene of the area and antibiotic therapy, particularly erythromycin, for 7 to 10 days.

Erysipelas

Erysipelas is an acute streptococcal skin infection that is a distinct and more superficial variant of cellulitis. Occurring most often in infants and middle-aged adults, lesions begin clinically as a red, localized area and spread rapidly with advancing, typically raised red margins. The disease usually affects the face and is associated with chills, fever, and marked toxicity. Edema of the affected area, often with bleb formation, may be prominent, and the eyes are frequently swollen shut. The infection may be transmitted to other individuals and, if contracted by dental personnel, will probably necessitate their absence from a dental practice for a few days. As in any streptococcal infection, complications may develop, such as scarring, spreading cellulitis, and even acute glomerulonephritis. Treatment is essentially antimicrobial, and penicillin is the drug of choice.

Bacterial Paronychia

Bacterial paronychial infections are relatively common in dental personnel. They are often due to a staphylococcal infection that produces a painful, red swelling of the soft tissue adjacent to the nail. Infections extending all the way around the nail bed are known as "runarounds." Drainage of pus, if required, may be accomplished by insertion of a sterile scalpel tip parallel to the nail plate. Systemic, rather than topical, antibiotic therapy is almost always indicated. Distinguishing between staphylococcal paronychia, herpetic paronychia, or paronychias caused by *Candida albicans* may be difficult, and microscopic smears or cultures of the lesion may be required.

Tenosynovitis

Tenosynovitis, an infection of the tendon sheath, may have serious sequelae for dentists. Dental personnel often develop tenosynovitis following a puncture or stab wound whereby a contaminated instrument or dental bur punctures a finger, hand, or forearm. This infection may be extremely serious because of its potential for rapid spread and possible destruction of the tendon sheath or tendon itself. Pain, functional interference, and induration may develop within a few hours after the injury. Healing is generally uneventful in injuries of this type; however, these injuries are not to be taken casually and should be treated promptly by appropriate antibiotic therapy and immobilization of the affected part.

Conjunctivitis

Conjunctivitis may occur rather readily in dental personnel who do not take proper precautions such as the wearing of eyeglasses or special protective eyewear. Conjunctivitis in the dental environment is usually due to bacteria or viruses entering the eye from contaminated oral aerosols, particles generated by rotary instruments, ultrasonic scalers, or air/water sprays. These conjunctival inflammations may do no more than create a reddened appearance to the conjunctiva or produce minor symptoms such as a dry, scratchy sensation or the feeling of a foreign body in the eye. The affected individual may notice some degree of photophobia, which may become more pronounced when visualizing the working area with the bright dental unit light or from fiberoptic devices. Unattended eye infections may lead to a purulent discharge with inability to open the eyelid and dried crust around the eyelids (Fig 3–1). Eye infections of any nature demand prompt attention by an ophthalmologist in view of the potentially serious consequences such as corneal scarring or impairment of vision. In addition to the wearing of protective eyewear by dental personnel, other preventive measures against eye infections include the use of the rubber dam and high-volume evacuation.

Tuberculosis

Historically, tuberculosis has been the most common cause of death throughout the world, accounting for 3 million deaths each year. Even today in the United States, tuberculosis remains the second leading cause of death related to infectious diseases. Approximately 15 million persons in this country have a positive tuberculin skin test indicating that infection with tubercle bacilli has occurred. Among this infected group, 90% will probably never develop active tuberculosis, but the remaining 10% will likely develop clinical tuberculosis at some time during their life. The predictions that tuberculosis would be essentially eradicated in the United States before the end of this century appear to be overly optimistic in view of the fact that 1 of every 4 men and 1 of every 5 women in this country still show evidence of exposure and sensitivity to tubercle bacilli.

The disease is caused by the *Mycobacterium tuberculosis* bacilli and is

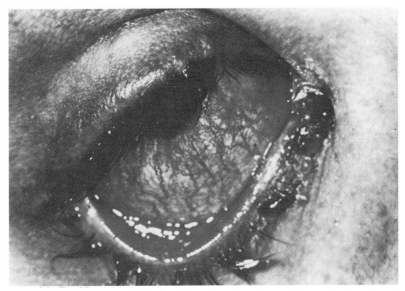

Fig 3–1.—Purulent eye infection in a dental student with marked conjunctival inflammation and crusting. Protective eyewear might have prevented this infection.

more prevalent among the poor, particularly those living with poor nutrition in crowded conditions. Predominantly an airborne disease, the contaminated droplets are discharged into the air by a person with active disease. These droplet nuclei may remain suspended in the air for a period of time, ready to be inhaled by a susceptible individual even after the infected person leaves the immediate area. Once the infected droplets fall onto the surface of an object, they cannot, for practical purposes, be aerosolized again and no longer represent a significant infectious hazard to most individuals. Thus, the outmoded practices that required special handling of the patient's bedclothes, dishes, and other fomites are no longer considered necessary.

When a nonimmune (susceptible) person inhales the tuberculosis bacilli, the organisms begin to slowly multiply at the site of deposition on the tiny air sacs (alveoli) of the lungs. The organisms continue to multiply and spread by lymphatic and hematogenous pathways to regional lymph nodes and other organs. Within a few days, the tubercle bacilli have disseminated to most parts of the body. About 4 to 8 weeks after infection, the individual develops "tuberculin hypersensitivity," an allergic reaction to the tuberculins. Significant tissue damage and necrosis may develop as a result of the allergic immune response of the host within weeks, months, or years after initiation of the infection in the 10% who are susceptible. The primary infection with tuberculosis provides immunity against subsequent bacilli that may be inhaled as droplet nuclei. Primary tuberculosis usually heals and the lesions become calcified, but if healing is imperfect or the immune system is incapable of containing and preventing growth of the tubercle bacilli, then active disease will result. If cavitating lesions develop in the lungs, these patients will spew incredible numbers of organisms into their air passages, which are then expelled as infected droplets into the air outside the body. These droplets could then infect another susceptible person, thus setting up a chain reaction of events.

There are usually few symptoms associated with primary tuberculosis. Any symptoms present soon disappear, and the infection enters a dormant stage. The active stage is typically insidious, with vague symptoms such as fatigue, cough, weight loss, fever or chills, nightsweats, states of nervous irritability, malaise, and loss of appetite. The more publicized symptoms of hemoptysis (spitting up of blood or blood-stained sputum) and chest pains are uncommon. Severe coughing is uncommon in the early disease stages, and shortness of breath does not usually occur until the lungs become extensively damaged. Tuberculosis may reactivate when an individual's immune system becomes impaired, thus allowing a recurring cycle of infection/disease/infection to occur.

Oral lesions of tuberculosis are uncommon despite the presence of a positive sputum in many patients. The tongue is the most frequent site of oral involvement, although lesions do occur on the lips, cheeks, palate, salivary glands, and even periapical regions (Fig 3–2). The oral lesions may begin as small tubercles that break down to form ulcers that are typically painful. There is no characteristic appearance for the oral lesions, and, like syphilis, tuberculosis can also be a great imitator of other diseases.

DIFFERENTIAL DIAGNOSIS.—In the clinical detection of oral lesions, diagnoses might include fungal diseases, syphilis, traumatic lesions, squamous cell carcinoma, and other infectious ulcers.

DETECTION OF TUBERCULOSIS.—This can be achieved by skin testing, chest x-ray, or examination and culture of sputum, pleural fluid, or gastric contents. Biopsy of oral lesions may be indicated. Skin testing plays an important role in large-scale screening programs, as demonstrated by the tine test and more accurately by the Mantoux test using a purified protein derivative (PPD) of the tubercle bacilli. One of the limitations of the skin test is that it makes no distinction between a person who is merely infected with tubercle bacilli and a person who has active disease. Every person who has a positive tuberculin skin test is at some risk (up to 10%) of developing active disease and should receive appropriate evaluation and possibly chemoprophylaxis.

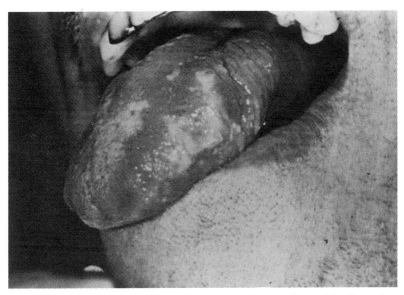

Fig 3–2.—Tuberculous ulcers on the tongue in a patient with disseminated tuberculosis.

TREATMENT OF TUBERCULOSIS.—Treatment is essentially chemotherapy, utilizing a variable drug regimen composed of isoniazid, rifampin, streptomycin, ethambutol, and several other drugs. At least two drugs are given simultaneously for control of active disease because of naturally occurring drug-resistant organisms developing from spontaneous mutation of tubercle bacilli. The administration of these drugs must be given over an adequate period of time ranging from 9 to 18 months. With proper chemotherapy, 90% of the patients with pulmonary tuberculosis should have negative cultures within 3 months. In persons who are being treated for active disease, monthly bacteriologic studies of the sputum are performed until the cultures are negative for growth of the tubercle bacilli. Treatment is continued for at least 6 months after the cultures become negative, and close follow-up of the patient is maintained for 1 year after completion of therapy to make sure relapse does not occur. Tuberculosis patients are subject to reactivation of their disease when poor health supervenes or their resistance becomes lowered.

It is now recognized that, with proper treatment, the tuberculosis victim does not have to be locked away in a sanitorium for the course of his disease. Tuberculosis is actually quite amenable to therapy, with a potential cure rate of 98% in patients receiving initial treatment. The patient does need to control his secretions, and the wearing of an effective mask by the patient will help control the air dispersal of organisms. During dental therapy, the patient with active disease will obviously be unable to wear a mask, and elective dental procedures on such patients with positive sputums should be postponed if possible. If urgent dental treatment is required, then the attending dental personnel should exercise every precaution in masking, gloving, and sterilization. Ideally, treatment of active disease patients should be performed in a special dental operatory set aside and equipped for the proper management of infectious disease patients.

It is important that dentists and their auxiliaries be skin tested annually or more often in the case of a known exposure or if symptoms develop. The potential for dental personnel to come in contact with patients who show evidence of previous exposure to tuberculosis is reasonably high (1 in 4 men and 1 in 5 women). Woodruff estimates that each year a dentist will see at least one unknown tuberculosis patient for an approximate incidence of one in every 1,500 patients. Those dentists working with Indochinese or Haitian refugees may wish to exercise additional precautions in their treatment in view of the increased incidence of several infectious diseases in these groups.

Fungal Infections

Dermatophytosis

Dental personnel may occasionally experience fungal skin infections, primarily of the fingers and hands. Frequent washing of the hands and working in a moist, contaminated environment may predispose one to develop superficial skin infections such as dermatophytosis and cutaneous candidiasis. Dermatophytosis, known also as ringworm or tinea, refers to mycotic infection of keratinized tissues such as nails, skin, or hair. Keeping the skin tightly covered for prolonged periods enhances susceptibility to superficial fungal infection. Skin reactions to dermatophytes are still not well understood, but may represent a response to toxins produced or a delayed hypersensitivity reaction. The symptoms of skin dermatophyte infection may vary from mild redness and itching to excoriation and pain. Mechanical deformities of the nails and hair may result from the digestion of keratin by fungal enzymes. The diagnosis of dermatophytosis may be suspected by physical examination and can be confirmed by microscopic examination and culturing of skin or nail scrapings. If left untreated, some dermatophytic infections may worsen and stubbornly persist, but in general, the proper use of certain antifungal agents is curative. Griseofulvin, an orally administered antibiotic with fungistatic effect, is the drug of choice for nail or hair infections. Fungistatic amounts are deposited in the keratin, which gradually exfoliates and is replaced by noninfected tissue. Treatment for infected fingernails may require 4 months or more of continuous griseofulvin therapy. Topical agents such as tolnaftate and the newer imidazole derivatives (miconazole and clotrimazole) in conjunction with hydrocortisone may also be used for effective treatment.

Candidiasis

Candidiasis of the skin is usually due to the yeast *C. albicans* and rarely to other *Candida* species. Like dermatophytosis, occlusion and maceration of the skin may be predisposing factors to infection. Underlying systemic diseases such as diabetes mellitus, hypoparathyroidism, or immune suppression may also be predisposing factors to infection by *Candida*.

The lesions of cutaneous candidiasis have a predilection for occurrence in intertriginous areas (beneath the breasts, axillae, groin, toe and finger webs) and the hands when they are immersed in water frequently or for extended periods. On the hands, the lesions may develop in the webs between the fingers and exhibit moist, pink surfaces with white, curd-like plaques at the periphery. Paronychial infections with candidiasis exhibit tenderness, redness, and swelling of the tissues around the nail. The tentative diagnosis is usually confirmed by microscopic examination and/or culturing of skin or nail samples (Fig 3–3). Treatment usually consists of topical application of antifungal agents such as nystatin, miconazole, clotrimazole, or ketoconazole.

Preventive measures for dental personnel include proper and careful

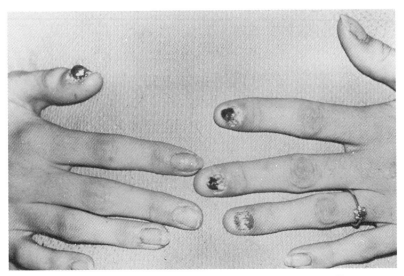

Fig 3–3.—Severe *C. albicans* infection of the fingernails.

drying of the hands after washing and trying to avoid immersing the hands for extended periods in water.

Fungal diseases in general do not appear to represent a significant occupational hazard for most healthy dental practitioners. Certain respiratory fungal diseases such as histoplasmosis, coccidioidomycosis, cryptococcosis, and blastomycosis do occur in dental personnel, but probably with no significant difference from the incidence in the general population for a given geographic location. The lack of adequate reporting and documentation of systemic fungal diseases in dental personnel leaves us with insufficient epidemiologic data to assess the problem.

Viral Infections

Hand, Foot, and Mouth Disease

Hand, foot, and mouth disease is a vesicular, ulcerative disease usually caused by a Coxsackie type A virus. The disease occurs most often in children under 10 years of age, is contagious, and tends to occur more often in the summer or late fall. Upon transmission of the virus by contact or droplet infection, a short incubation period of 3 to 5 days may be followed by vague initial symptoms such as sore throat, malaise, and fever. These initial symptoms may occur 24 to 48 hours prior to the development of skin or oral lesions. The oral lesions are usually the first clinical sign of the disease and initially appear as bright red macules on the tongue, gingiva, or other intraoral sites. A short-lived vesicular stage of the initial lesion is followed by the formation of shallow, yellow-to-gray ulcerations with erythematous halos. The oral lesions are painful, but resolve in 7 to 10 days. The cutaneous lesions of the hand and foot may also be painful and are located on the sides of the fingers or toes and borders of the palms or soles. The skin lesions appear as red papules aligned in a linear fashion often paralleling the skin lines and usually resolve within 2 weeks. Occasionally, lesions on the extremities do not develop, but oral lesions are always present. The clinical differential diagnosis of the oral lesions might include herpetic gingivostomatitis, recurrent aphthous ulcers, herpangina, and erythema multiforme. Detection of hand, foot, and mouth disease rests primarily upon the clinician's recognition of the distribution of lesions. Viral cultures can be performed (usually on fecal specimens) for positive identification, but this is not usually warranted. Treatment is basically supportive and symptomatic, because this self-limiting disease usually runs its course within 2 weeks.

Hand, foot, and mouth disease is of importance to dentists because of the contagious nature of the disease and the possibility that the exposed dentist could transmit the disease to other patients, office personnel, and family. During the active stage of early clinical lesions, an infected dentist should attempt to restrict his contacts with people and, ideally, refrain from direct patient care for a few days.

Herpes Simplex

There are more than 70 types of herpes viruses known to produce disease in animals; however, only five of these are known to affect humans. These are the DNA-containing herpes viruses (HSV) Type 1 and Type 2, the Epstein-Barr virus (EBV), the varicella-zoster virus (VZV), and the cytomegalovirus (CMV). For years, investigators have attempted to implicate the herpes viruses in the induction of human cancer. For example, HSV-1 and EBV have been suggested as etiologic agents in nasopharyngeal carcinoma, and HSV-2 infection in women is associated with an increased risk of cervical carcinoma. Herpes infections are of great practical importance to dentists, because herpetic lesions of the finger or eye may produce temporary inability to practice. Repeated recurrences of ocular herpes can lead to blindness and permanent inability to practice.

Although less than 1% of the population has a history of clinically evident HSV-1 primary oral infection, it is estimated that up to 80% of adults in the lower socioeconomic groups in the United States have HSV-1 antibodies, whereas only 30% to 50% of adults in the higher socioeconomic groups have these antibodies to demonstrate previous herpetic infection. Thus, it appears that the frequency of previous herpetic infection is inversely related to socioeconomic status. In a study conducted by Rowe and coworkers, the prevalence of herpes virus was found to increase with age among dentists. Their research indicates that dental students (since they tend to come from middle- or high-income families) and young dentists are less likely to have previous experience with herpetic infection and may be more susceptible to developing primary herpes virus infections as adults. This study revealed some very interesting and somewhat unexpected findings in that the frequency of herpes labialis and herpetic eye infections occurred less often in dentists than in the control population. Conversely, it was found that herpetic whitlow (paronychia) occurred twice as frequently in practicing dentists as in the control population.

The herpes simplex viruses (HSV-1 and HSV-2) will usually infect epithelial cells. Normally, HSV-1 affects the oral and pharyngeal regions, while HSV-2 affects the genital region. This division of site-specificity (for HSV-1 to occur above the waist and for HSV-2 to occur below the waist) is becoming less apparent to some extent because of the change in sexual practices with more interchange between oral and genital regions. It has been estimated that 5% of primary herpetic gingivostomatitis infections in adults are due to HSV-2 and that up to 15% of genital herpes infections may be associated with HSV-1. There are no distinguishing features to allow accurate clinical differentiation of HSV-1 from HSV-2 infections in the mouth or oropharynx; neither does there appear to be a marked difference in their clinical behavior, although a few investigators have voiced the opinion that HSV-2 infections in the oral cavity take somewhat longer to resolve.

Primary oral herpes infections usually occur in young children (6 months to 5 years of age) approximately 4 to 10 days following exposure of a seronegative individual to the infectious viral particle. Spread of the virus by direct contact is probably the most common mode of exposure, although the fecal-oral route of spread may be of some importance. The initial manifestations of the oral herpes infection may be fever, restlessness, and irritability. Oral lesions usually appear 1 to 4 days later in the form of a diffuse gingivitis, which is often marginal (band-like) in type, and a widespread eruption of vesicles on the oral or pharyngeal mucosa. The vesicles in primary herpetic gingivostomatitis rupture soon after they appear to leave small punctate ulcers often surrounded by a well-defined red halo. The lesions may coalesce to form large ulcers, but usually heal without scarring in 14 to 21 days. Primary herpetic gingivostomatitis may also be seen in adults (usually young adults), and here the infection may be more severe than in children (Fig 3–4). Following an infection, the virus will assume a state of latency, and studies suggest that the oral herpes simplex virus travels back along nerve fibers to the sensory nerve ganglia of the second and third division of the trigeminal nerve. Here the virus remains latent until reactivated by nonspecific stimuli and then travels back along the peripheral nerves to the epithelial surface to produce subclinical or clinical recurrent infection. Recurrent forms of oral herpes include recurrent intraoral herpes and herpes labialis (cold sores). Recurrent intraoral herpes tends to affect mucosa overlying bone (hard palate, alveolar ridge), while herpes labialis is usually located on the outer vermillion border of the lips and perioral skin surfaces. Recurrent infections are generally less severe and typically reappear in the same location. Recurrent lesions may develop only sporadically; however, monthly recurrences are not uncommon in some unfortunate individuals. Periodic reactivation of the herpes virus occurs in at least one half of infected persons, with great variation in the frequency and duration of recurrent lesions.

LABORATORY ASSISTANCE.—In the diagnosis of intraoral herpes infections, treatment is not always essential, because the clinical features are often reasonably diagnostic. However, confirmation in doubtful cases may be indicated, and the aspiration of a vesicle, cytologic smear of an ulcer, viral culture, or biopsy of a representative lesion can all produce acceptable

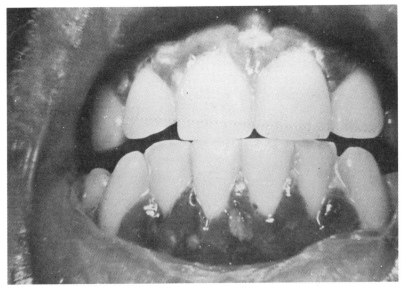

Fig 3–4.—Primary herpetic gingivostomatitis in a young adult. Clinical differentiation between HSV-1 and HSV-2 infection is impractical if not impossible.

material for microscopic diagnosis. The cytologic smears need to be obtained early in the disease, preferably during the vesicular stage or soon after the vesicles rupture. For a viral culture, the specimen obtained should be placed in a virus transport medium (i.e., VTM-Gibco Biocult) and sent to the laboratory as quickly as possible. The viral culture is not often indicated for oral herpes infection because of the logistics, time, and expense required to obtain results. When available, electron microscopy is another useful laboratory procedure to assist in the identification of a virus. A rapid immunofluorescence test and an immunoperoxidase test with good sensitivity and specificity have been developed, but they are not yet widely available. A number of serologic techniques ranging from the older methods of precipitation to the newer radioimmunoassay (RIA) and enzyme-linked immunoabsorbent assay (ELISA) are now available. Serum samples from the patient in the acute and convalescent stages of the disease can be evaluated for antibody titer to the herpes simplex virus. A fourfold increase in HSV antibody titer is indicative of a primary infection, while a much smaller rise in antibody titer is seen with recurrent HSV infections.

CLINICAL DIFFERENTIAL DIAGNOSIS.—Intraoral herpes simplex infections might include the diagnoses of aphthous ulcers; herpangina; hand, foot, and mouth disease; herpes zoster; and erythema multiforme.

TREATMENT.—Treatment of intraoral herpes lesions remains basically supportive. Herpes labialis patients may benefit from the topical application of antiviral agents such as 5-iodo-2-deoxyuridine (IDU), cytosine arabinoside (Ara-C), adenine arabinoside (Ara-A), or acyclovir. Some affected individuals report fewer recurrences or decreased severity of recurrent infection from the daily ingestion of lysine (300 to 1,400 mg/day) or citrus bioflavonoids and vitamin C. The use of corticosteroids to treat herpetic lesions is best avoided and should only be used in special circumstances. Fortunately, the great majority of herpetic infections encountered by the dentist are self-limiting and usually resolve within 3 weeks.

Herpetic Whitlow (Paronychia)

It was not recognized until 1959 that a primary herpetic infection could occur on the fingers of adults. Herpetic paronychia (felon) is a common affliction among dental and medical personnel. Usually inoculation occurs through direct contact with a herpetic lesion or through saliva containing herpes simplex virus. Autoinfection may also occur, such as in individuals who are nail biters and have the virus in their saliva. At 3 to 7 days after inoculation of the finger, the patient may notice intense pain, swelling, and the formation of vesicles near the injury site (Fig 3–5). The infection often affects the index finger or thumb of dentists, and the pain may be so excruciating as to prevent the individual from practicing dentistry. The infection typically localizes to one finger, but may spread to adjacent sites. Vesicles frequently develop on the finger pad and coalesce (Fig 3–6). Regional lymph nodes may become enlarged and tender in the arm or axilla, and a low-grade fever may be present. At 3 to 4 weeks after the injury, the lesions are usually healed, but recurrence is a likely possibility. The pain and incapacitation associated with herpetic paronychia in the early stages is well appreciated by those individuals stricken with this occupational hazard.

Treatment is essentially isolation of the involved finger, limitation of movement of the involved site, refrain from rubbing or scratching lesion to prevent spread, and analgesics as required. Preventive measures include the wearing of gloves, attempt to prevent self-injury of the hands, and the reappointment of any patient who has obvious vesicular-stage lesions that suggest herpes simplex virus.

Ocular Herpes

Herpes simplex infections of the eye are usually caused by HSV-1, although HSV-2 is occasionally recovered from the eye. The primary infection is usually a conjunctivitis and sometimes an associated keratitis. The fact that an individual has already had an oral HSV-1 infection does not

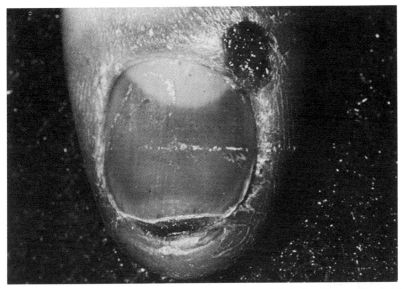

Fig 3–5.—Seven-day-old herpetic whitlow on the left index finger. Dentist inoculated his finger with a contaminated instrument while treating a patient with recurrent herpes labialis.

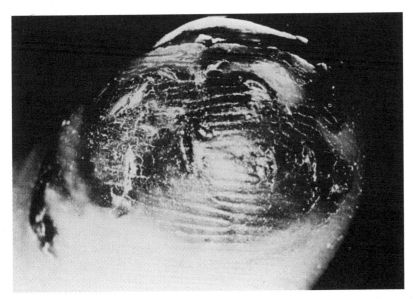

Fig 3–6.—Eighteen-day-old nerpetic whitlow in the left index finger of a periodontist. Multiple vesicles coalesced to form a large, painful lesion. At 35 days, the lesion was relatively well healed.

necessarily prevent the development of an eye or genital herpetic infection. Recurrences of herpetic keratitis of the cornea are common, whereas recurrent conjunctivitis is less common. Herpetic keratitis may temporarily prevent the dentist from practicing because of painful ulcers and visual impairment. Recurrent herpetic keratitis may lead to progressive scarring, opacification of the cornea, and even permanent visual damage. In fact, herpes infection of the cornea is the most common infectious disease causing blindness in this country.

Herpes infections of the eye should be evaluated by an ophthalmologist, and treatment is principally the topical application of antiviral agents. Preventive measures include the wearing of protective eyewear and measures to reduce the formation of contaminated oral aerosols.

Routine treatment of patients with primary acute herpetic gingivostomatitis should be delayed until the clinical symptoms have disappeared. Emergency treatment requiring extraction or tissue manipulation could result in increased patient discomfort and severity of infection. Herpes simplex infections pose fewer problems for the patient and the dentist if routine preventive measures are observed.

Hepatitis

Viral hepatitis is a disease of global importance from the standpoint of morbidity, mortality, and economic impact from the millions of man-hours lost as a result of this disease each year. In the United States, forms of viral hepatitis occur in hundreds of thousands of individuals each year. There are at least three known forms of viral hepatitis: the hepatitis A virus (HAV), the hepatitis B virus (HBV), and the non-A, non-B hepatitis virus (NANB). Hepatitis B is of the utmost importance to members of the dental profession in view of their past and present exposure to this serious disease. Dentists surveyed at the American Dental Association annual session in 1972 revealed that about 13% of those evaluated had a history of exposure to HBV. From 1975 to 1980, the American Dental Association survey revealed that 28% of dentists had previous hepatitis experience. This rate is equivalent to the highest rates of exposure in the medical profession among surgeons and pathologists. Whether or not this reflects an increased incidence of HBV in dentists or heightened awareness with more accurate reporting and testing is not presently known. The HBV risk in general dentists is three times that of the general population, while the risk for oral surgeons and periodontists is up to ten times that of the general population. Estimates of the average incidence of the HBV carrier state in the general population of this country range from 0.1% to 0.5%. Dentists as a group may have up to ten times the normal risk of developing the HBV carrier state.

HAV

Formerly referred to as "infectious hepatitis," HAV has an incubation period of 2 to 6 weeks, with the average period being about 28 days. The HAV is an RNA-containing virus usually transmitted through fecal contamination of water or food, although it can be transmitted in saliva. The fecal-oral route of infection may infect an entire household or create an epidemic in institutions with poor sanitation and overcrowding. The disease is usually abrupt in onset and occurs more often in children, although an increasing number of adults are being reported with HAV. Fever is noted often (50% to 70% of patients), but is uncommon in the other types of viral hepatitis. Other constitutional symptoms for any form of acute viral hepatitis may include headache, fatigue, skin rash, arthralgia, and nonspecific gastrointestinal and respiratory symptoms. Jaundice may or may not develop, although dark brown urine and clay-colored stools may be noted a few days before jaundice (the icteric stage) develops. As clinical jaundice appears, the prodromal symptoms usually diminish. The HAV typically has the shortest convalescent stage, because clinical recovery occurs more rapidly in this form of viral hepatitis. A chronic-carrier state does not develop in HAV, and the mortality rate is less than 0.5%.

HBV

Hepatitis B is due to a 42-nm double-shell DNA virus originally known as the Dane particle. The disease occurs most often in 15- to 30-year-old individuals, accounts for up to 50% of cases of fulminant viral hepatitis, and may have a mortality rate of 1%. Approximately 200,000 cases of HBV occur each year in the United States, and nearly a fourth of these individuals will develop acute disease with jaundice. The now-discarded term of "serum hepatitis" is a misnomer, because it is now known that HBV can be spread by more avenues than blood or blood products. Many body secretions such as saliva, semen, bile, vaginal secretions, milk, and even urine can contain the HBV surface antigen (HBsAg) and are theoretically capable of transmitting the disease. The amount of viral particles produced in a patient with HBV is phenomenal and can result in 10^6 to 10^7 viral particles per milliliter of blood. This extremely high titer of virus requires only minute amounts (one ten-thousandth of a milliliter) of contaminated blood or small amounts of other infected body secretions to transmit enough virus to produce disease in a susceptible person. Transmission of the virus in dental personnel is primarily by contaminated blood or saliva through a break in the skin of the hands (percutaneous route) or possibly through the mucous membranes (permucosal route) of the eyes, mouth, or nose. The role played by blood or saliva splashed into the permucosal routes is probably much smaller and less efficient than the percutaneous route through a minor wound of the fingers or hands. Air transmission of HBV through inhalation of contaminated blood does not appear to be a likely hazard for dental personnel, because blood is not aerosolized well. Infected blood, saliva, and other body fluids may contaminate and survive for days on surfaces such as counter tops, dental unit switches, and other environmental surfaces in the dental operatory. How important this is as a risk factor is difficult to assess, because there is little evidence that the virus can withstand routine cleaning or disinfection of these surfaces.

The incubation period for HBV may be relatively long, with 6 weeks to 6 months elapsing before clinical symptoms develop. The onset and severity of the disease may be dose-dependent, with large viral inocula tending to have a shorter incubation period and the more likely development of acute icteric HBV. An insidious onset with prolonged prodromal manifestations such as malaise and arthralgia is more likely in HBV than in HAV. An affected individual may notice early symptoms such as easy fatigability, requirement for more rest and sleep, and frequent headaches. A serum sickness-like syndrome with joint pain, fever, and/or a maculopapular skin rash occurs in 10% to 20% of the cases with acute HBV (Fig 3–7). Other symptoms, including anorexia, nausea, vomiting, abdominal pain, severe fatigue, depression, darkening of the urine, liver tenderness, clay-colored stools, and finally jaundice, may all occur in the icteric form of this disease. In contrast, another affected individual may have a subclinical infection with mild symptoms that go relatively unnoticed.

Development of the chronic-carrier state occurs in 5% to 10% of acute HBV cases, whereas HAV is not known to produce a chronic-carrier state. The chronic-carrier state in HBV is exhibited by the persistence of HBsAg in the blood. The carrier state is more likely to occur in the 50% or more of HBV patients who do not develop clinical signs of jaundice in the anicteric disease form, but who may have prolonged low-grade symptoms and mild serum biochemical abnormalities. This paradoxic finding produces chronic carriers of HBsAg who frequently have no recollection of acute HBV symptoms. About half of the initial carriers of HBsAg will eliminate the virus within 2 years, whereas the other half will remain in the carrier state for months to years or indefinitely. More than 170 million people in the world today are believed to be chronically infected with HBV. In the United States, the Centers for Disease Control estimate that there are up to 1 million chronic carriers, and this number increases 2% to 3% annually. The largest human reservoir of HBV is found in chronic carriers. Consequently, it is this unknown carrier of HBV that poses the greatest threat to all health care workers, because there are no readily identifiable clinical features that allow for their recognition and subsequent precautions for treatment.

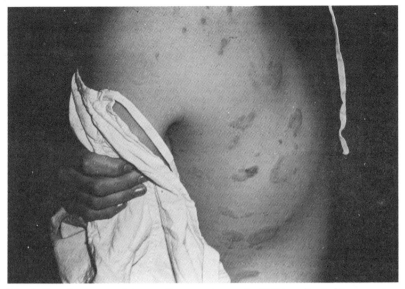

Fig 3–7.—A serum sickness-like syndrome in HBV patient. The syndrome may be an early manifestation and can consist of skin rash, joint pain, and fever.

Non-A, Non-B Hepatitis

Infection with NANB is the most common cause of posttransfusion hepatitis in 90% to 95% of cases. Approximately 230,000 new cases of NANB related to blood transfusion occur in this country each year. It is principally a type of viral hepatitis diagnosed by exclusion in that there are currently no specific serologic tests available for NANB virus(es). The diagnosis is made most often after the exclusion of HAV or HBV by negative serologic tests. The clinical symptoms may be particularly mild or absent inasmuch as two thirds of the reported cases have few or no apparent symptoms. Development of the chronic-carrier state occurs much more commonly than with HBV. Little is known at present about the development of serious sequelae such as carcinoma of the liver, but there is an expected mortality rate in this disease of up to 1%.

Laboratory Tests

Laboratory tests for the detection of viral hepatitis are based principally on serodiagnostic techniques. Specific antigens and antibodies can be detected in blood and other biologic fluids that follow a predictable serologic pattern during the course of HAV or HBV infection. For serodiagnosis of HAV, demonstration of IgM antibody against HAV (IgM anti-HAV) is indicative of recent infection and is detectable for at least 4 to 6 months after illness begins. A second antibody, IgG anti-HAV, which is also specific for the HAV antigen, appears after the acute illness and generally remains detectable for a lifetime. At least 30% of our general population demonstrates this antibody to indicate previous exposure to HAV.

As early as 3 to 4 weeks after infection, HBsAg may begin to appear, and this may precede biochemical changes or symptoms by 2 to 4 weeks (Fig 3–8, Table 3–1). The HBV e antigen (HBeAg) appears along with HBsAg before symptoms develop, and the most infectious period is during the short-lived presence of HBeAg. Antibody to HBV core antigen (Anti-HBc) appears around the time symptoms are noticed. It is useful in documenting a recent acute infection during the so-called "window" period when the normal immune response has practically eliminated surface antigens with surface antibody. During this convalescence window, the amounts of surface antibody present are too small to be detected. Detection of antibody to HBV e antigen (Anti-HBe) during the acute stage signals a favorable prognosis that complete resolution of the infection is likely. Finally, neutralizing antibody against HBsAg (Anti-HBs) appears 12 to 16 weeks after the onset of symptoms and follows the disappearance of HBsAg. The presence of Anti-HBs indicates immunologic recovery from HBV and provides long-lasting protection against HBV upon reexposure to the virus. If HBsAg and HBeAg persist for longer than 10 weeks, this may indicate that a chronic-carrier state is developing. These patients should be periodically monitored to see if possible seroconversion to antibody formation occurs.

TABLE 3–1.—SEROLOGIC MARKERS FOR HEPATITIS B VIRUS INFECTION

SEROLOGIC MARKER	DEFINITION AND DESCRIPTION
HBsAg	HBV surface antigen. Usually the earliest serologic marker detected. May precede symptoms and biochemical changes by 2 to 4 weeks. Persistence may be indicative of chronic-carrier state.
HBeAg	HBV e antigen. Appears in serum shortly after HBsAg. Is an early indicator of acute active infection and period of highest infectivity. Persistence longer than 10 weeks may indicate development of carrier state and chronic liver disease.
Anti-HBc	Antibody to HBV core antigen. Appears in serum after HBsAg and is another indicator of acute infection. May be only serologic marker detectable during "convalescence window" period between disappearance of HBsAg and before Anti-HBs appears.
Anti-HBe	Antibody to HBV e antigen. Loss of e antigen through seroconversion to e antibody in acute stage indicates probable recovery and resolution of infection.
Anti-HBs	Antibody to HBV surface antigen. Indicates immunologic recovery from infection and immunity against reinfection. Ordinarily appears in serum 3 to 4 months after initial symptoms, but may be delayed.

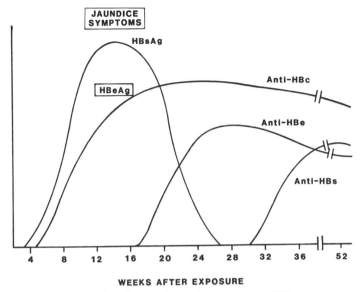

Fig 3–8.—Serologic markers in acute HBV.

Other laboratory tests can be used to demonstrate biochemical abnormalities in hepatitis. Liver function tests, including the serum transaminases (SGOT, SGPT) and others, will be elevated during active disease, indicating damage of the liver cells.

Treatment Measures

There is no specific treatment for any form of acute viral hepatitis once the infection develops; however, there are prophylactic measures for HAV and HBV. Pooled gamma globulin (immune serum globulin or ISG) can be up to 85% effective in the prevention of HAV, but its efficacy in HBV prophylaxis is inconclusive. Hepatitis B immune globulin (hyperimmune globulin or HBIG) has been generally adopted as the method of choice for treating needle-sticks or other acute exposure situations of HBV in health care workers. Because it is obtained from donors who have higher titers of HBV surface antibody than is found among pooled gamma globulin donors, HBIG should afford a higher level of prophylactic protection when given soon after exposure. However, HBIG is expensive, and recent studies have recommended that either agent can be used for postexposure prophylaxis following parenteral exposure to HBV. The administration of ISG or HBIG provides only passive immunization with a variable degree of success in preventing disease in the exposed individual. Active immunization with an approved commercial vaccine (Heptavax-B by Merck, Sharp, and Dohme) became available in mid-1982. The HBV vaccine is derived from the plasma of chronic carriers and is highly effective in promoting neutralizing antibody (Anti-HBs) formation. The vaccine may provide active immunity against HBV in 80% to 95% of the susceptible individuals. The vaccine is administered in three intramuscular doses, with one dose given initially, repeated at 1 month, and again at 6 months. The manufacturer is now working to develop a one-shot vaccine to provide the same level of protection. The vaccine appears to be very safe, with side effects being primarily mild constitutional symptoms as well as soreness and redness at the injection site. The actual length of protection and subsequent need for booster doses are not yet known, although available data suggest that immunity may last for 5 years or longer in patients who receive three doses of the vaccine. Although several subtypes of HBV exist, infection or immunization with one subtype provides immunity to all other subtypes. The vaccine has maximum effectiveness in nonexposed individuals and will not have a therapeutic effect in chronic HBV carriers, in persons who already have immunity against HBV, in HAV, or NANB viral infection. Proven recommendations for use of the vaccine in conjunction with HBIG or ISG for postexposure prophylaxis to HBV are not available at this time.

Sequelae

The sequelae and serious complications of HBV include the chronic-carrier state, massive liver necrosis, cirrhosis, chronic active hepatitis, and cancer of the liver. Approximately 4,000 deaths from cirrhosis associated with chronic HBV infection occur each year in this country. Chronic carriers of HBsAg are at a much greater risk (up to 273 times) of developing primary carcinoma of the liver. The recovery of some affected individuals may be lengthy and extend over a period of many months, with fatigue and lack of endurance being common complaints. Many recuperating dentists have noted that they were unable to endure the physical and mental rigors of a busy practice as they once could, even though 6 months or more had elapsed since the acute stage of their disease.

Preventive Measures

Preventive measures for dental personnel include appropriate precautions in the handling of blood, saliva, or other body secretions that are known to be contaminated with HBV and in working with high-risk groups of patients who are more likely to have or to carry HBV infection. Patient groups that are considered to present a higher incidence of HBV infection or the carrier state include, but are not limited to, the listing contained in Table 3–2.

TABLE 3–2.—PATIENT GROUPS AT INCREASED
RISK OF TRANSMITTING HBV

Low Risk:
   Health care workers with infrequent blood contact
Intermediate Risk:
   Male prisoners
   Health care workers with frequent blood contact
High Risk:
   Haitian or Indochinese refugees
   Drug addicts using parenteral drugs
   Homosexual males
   Hemodialysis patients
   Patients receiving multiple transfusions or blood
      products
   Some hematology or oncology patients
   Institutionalized mentally handicapped
   Intimate or household contacts of HBV carriers

The infectivity of saliva in the transmission of HBV has been questioned by some investigators; however, HBsAg is readily detectable in the saliva and must be considered a likely potential source of infection. Even saliva that is negative for occult blood can contain HBV that could conceivably come from the crevicular fluid of the gingival sulcus. Studies to confirm this and the possibility that the virus is secreted directly through the salivary glands are pending. How the virus enters the mouth—through occult blood, crevicular fluid, or saliva—is merely academic to the dentist and his coworkers.

The risk of developing clinical HBV following percutaneous or permucosal exposure to blood known to contain HBsAg is approximately 1:20, whereas if the antigen status in the blood is unknown, the risk is greatly reduced to about 1:2,000. Not everyone who has the HBsAg is transmitting the disease, and dentists or dental auxiliaries who show positive testing results for HBsAg should not despair. The biologic factors that cause some HBsAg carriers to be actual spreaders of the disease are not known, although there is some evidence to show that blood containing the HBeAg is more likely to be infective. In general, dentists are much more likely to contract HBV from their patients than they are to spread the disease to their patients. The "carrier dentist," whose serum test results are positive for the HBsAg, is faced with the moral and medical-legal issues pertaining to whether he must exercise informed consent. This would require the dentist to inform his patients of the low potential risk for transmission of his disease to them. This risk is greatly minimized by strict compliance with routine infection control procedures. The prudent asymptomatic carrier dentist should be able to continue his practice if he adheres to a strict regimen of preventive measures. This individual is advised to wear rubber gloves (preferably double gloves), a face mask, and attempt to conduct his practice in as sterile a manner as is possible to avoid every chance of his transmitting the disease to a patient. Thus far, there have been only isolated outbreaks where a dentist has transmitted HBV to a number of patients. Once a dentist is known to have transmitted HBV to a patient, he may run the risk of being liable in his future practice. In addition, there is the possibility that the dentist may experience some difficulty in obtaining adequate malpractice insurance coverage at a reasonable fee.

The dental profession has already been made aware of an alarmingly high rate of exposure to HBV, and it must accept the fact that the disease is developing in another 3% to 5% of susceptible dentists each year. When the consequences of possible death, long-term disability, carrier status, or risk of hepatocellular carcinoma are considered, the availability of an effective, safe vaccine should be strongly considered as a prophylactic measure for all dental personnel who do not have existing immunity against this disease.

Acquired Immune Deficiency Syndrome (AIDS)

This relatively new and inadequately understood condition is associated with an impairment in the body's immune system. Since 1978, a group of diseases associated with a specific defect in cell-mediated immunity has been recognized as manifested by Kaposi's sarcoma, *Pneumocystis carinii* pneumonia, *Toxoplasma gondii* infections, and other life-threatening opportunistic infections. The disease is typically accompanied by a change in the ratio between T-suppressor cells and T-helper cells with suppression predominating. Persons who have been found to be primarily at risk are homosexual men, intravenous drug users, Haitian immigrants, and hemophiliacs. Although the number of reported cases to date is only 2,500, the numbers are increasing rapidly, and the true extent of the problem is not yet known. Symptoms of AIDS include marked fatigue, persistent fevers or night sweats, weight loss unrelated to diet or activity, lymph node enlargement, discolored nodules on the skin or mucous membranes (particularly the mouth), persistent dry cough, and diarrhea. The victim may develop severe *Candida* and herpes infections of the mouth, skin, or anorectal area. Cytomegalovirus and HBV infection are frequently reported. Slightly more than one third of the AIDS patients to date have vascular neoplastic lesions (i.e., Kaposi's sarcoma of the mouth, skin, or lymphoid tissues) with or without concurrent *Pneumocystis* pneumonia, while two thirds have opportunistic infections without Kaposi's sarcoma.

The etiology of the underlying immune deficiencies seen in AIDS cases is unknown. However, one hypothesis consistent with current observations is that a transmissible agent may be involved. A number of viruses, including herpesviruses, human T-cell leukemia virus, cytomegalovirus, and EBV have been suggested as possible causes. The patterns of spread of the disease resemble the distribution and modes of spread of HBV, and HBV infections occur very frequently among AIDS cases.

There is presently little convincing evidence of AIDS transmission to hospital or dental personnel from contact with infected patients or clinical specimens. Nevertheless, because of concern about a possible transmissible agent, such personnel would be wise to use the same precautions when caring for patients with AIDS as those used for patients with HBV infection, in which blood and body fluids are considered potentially infective. Specifically, precautions should be taken to avoid direct contact of skin and mucous membranes with blood products, excretions, secretions, and tissues of persons judged likely to have AIDS.

Treatment for AIDS patients is difficult, because they often have multiple opportunistic infections requiring multiple drug therapy. For some infections, there are only a limited number of drugs available for effective treatment at this time, and some of these may not be safe for extensive use in humans. Mortality rates for AIDS victims are high, with death resulting in 20% who have Kaposi's sarcoma without *Pneumocystis* pneumonia as compared with a 67% death rate in patients who have both Kaposi's sarcoma and *Pneumocystis* pneumonia. Recent information released from the Centers for Disease Control revealed 852 deaths in 2,157 cases for an interim mortality rate of 39%. The death rate in the CDC cases is expected to increase with time and one AIDS treatment center reports no survivors 3 years after the onset of AIDS.

Venereal Infections

Syphilis

Syphilis has become the third-most-common reported infectious disease in the United States. *Treponema pallidum*, the causative spirochetal organism, is transmitted either by intimate contact with lesions of primary or secondary syphilis or from mother to the unborn child. Syphilis is classically described as a disease that occurs in three stages; however, these stages are not always clearly defined in a given patient with the disease.

The primary stage of syphilis usually develops within 3 weeks following intimate contact with an infected individual, but the incubation period may be as short as 10 days or as long as 90 days after contact. The initial lesion is called a chancre and is usually found in the genital region. Extragenital chancres may occur in 10% of the cases, and the finding of an intraoral chancre is not rare. There is no typical appearance for an intraoral chancre;

it may vary from an eroded papule to a deep ulceration. The chancre is usually solitary and is often located on the lips, but may be discovered on the tongue and other intraoral sites (Fig 3–9). The lesion may be somewhat painful, although it is not usually exquisitely symptomatic unless secondarily infected. Genital chancres are typically accompanied by a painless enlargement of regional lymph nodes, but oral chancres are occasionally associated with painful enlarged cervical or submandibular lymph nodes. The serologic tests for syphilis may be reactive or nonreactive in the primary stage, depending upon the duration of the disease. If treated properly with antibiotic therapy, the chancre may heal within a week, but even without therapy, it will heal in 4 to 6 weeks.

The secondary stage of syphilis develops after an interval of 4 to 10 weeks or more after disappearance of the primary stage, but in some cases secondary lesions appear while the chancre is still present. The secondary stage of syphilis is the most contagious because of the multiplicity of lesions that may develop on skin or mucous membrane. Over 80% of the patients with secondary syphilis will develop skin or mucous membrane lesions. Serologic tests for syphilis are reactive in essentially all secondary-stage patients. Mild systemic symptoms, including fever, malaise, headache, anorexia, sore throat, and lymphadenopathy, may precede or accompany the secondary stage. The skin lesions usually consist of a pink-to-red macular

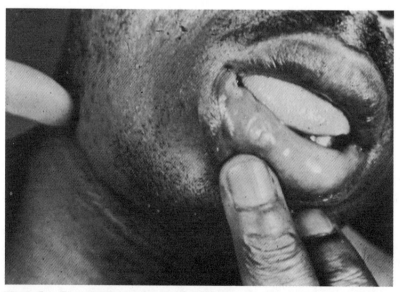

Fig 3–9.—Extragenital syphilitic chancres on the lower lip. Note presence of two ulcerative lesions on labial mucosa and enlarged right cervical lymph nodes.

or papular eruption that may be generalized, symmetric, and nonpruritic. The eruption varies greatly, but papulosquamous lesions of the palms and soles are characteristic, as is alopecia of the spotty type. The skin eruption usually heals without scarring in 2 to 10 weeks, but may persist for months unless therapy is instituted. The most infectious lesions in secondary syphilis are the moist lesions such as the mucous patches and the condyloma latum. Mucous patches may develop in the anogenital region, mouth, or throat. The intraoral mucous patch usually occurs on the lips, labial commissure (split papule), tongue, palate, or other regions. The mucous patch is a gray-white ulceration often surrounded by a red areola and is usually asymptomatic or only mildly symptomatic.

DIFFERENTIAL DIAGNOSIS.—Diagnoses of primary and secondary syphilitic oral lesions might include aphthous ulcers, traumatic and nonspecific ulcers, erythema multiforme, candidiasis, and herpetic lesions.

Latent syphilis may then develop in some untreated or inadequately treated patients and over a period of 10 to 20 years produce tertiary lesions such as syphilitic glossitis, gumma formation, and lesions in the central nervous system, and cardiovascular system.

LABORATORY TESTS.—Tests for the detection of syphilis include darkfield examination and serodiagnosis. Darkfield examination consists of the direct examination of infectious material from a primary or secondary lesion for the presence of spirochetal organisms. This test is useful for genital lesions, but has little application for saliva-contaminated oral lesions. Certain spirochetal organisms such as *Treponema microdentium* are a normal oral inhabitant and may closely simulate the appearance of *T. pallidum* on a darkfield examination. Serodiagnosis consists of two basic types: (1) nontreponemal antigens such as the venereal disease research laboratory test (VDRL) and (2) *T. pallidum* antigen tests such as the fluorescent treponemal antibody absorbed test (FTA-ABS) or the microhemagglutination *T. pallidum* test (MHA-TP).

TREATMENT.—Penicillin remains the drug of choice, and overall, the prognosis for syphilis is good if treated early. Delayed diagnosis and therapy may worsen the prognosis in bringing about seronegativity and developing late complications that are not as responsive to therapy.

The incidence of accidentally acquired syphilis is higher in dentists than in any other professional group. Chancres usually affect the left hand, particularly the fingertips, of dentists, and paronychia should arouse the suspicion of syphilis in every dentist. In general, syphilitic paronychias are less painful than those caused by bacterial or viral infection.

PREVENTIVE MEASURES.—For dental personnel, these simply consist of wearing rubber gloves, particularly in the presence of minor wounds or abrasions on the hands, and using common sense in examining suspicious lesions. These simple measures could totally prevent dental personnel from acquiring this disease through their hands.

Gonorrhea

Gonorrhea is the most commonly reported venereal disease, with the Centers for Disease Control estimating that in excess of 2½ million cases are treated each year in the United States. This means that one new case of gonorrhea occurs every 12 seconds. Metropolitan centers report the highest rates of gonococcal infection, with the highest incidence occurring among young adults (20 to 24 years of age), followed by teenagers (15 to 19 years of age).

Gonorrhea is an infectious, contagious disease caused by a gram-negative intracellular diplococcus, *Neisseria gonorrhoeae*. The infection is almost always transmitted through some form of sexual contact, although rarely it may occur by contact with freshly contaminated articles such as instruments and other inanimate objects. Asymptomatic carriers of both sexes constitute the reservoir of gonococcal infection that may be spread throughout the community. Estimates of the frequency of asymptomatic carriers range from 50% to 70% of infected women and 15% to 35% of infected men.

Oral and pharyngeal regions are common extragenital sites in which the primary lesions in these areas are usually located as a result of some direct form of oral sex, primarily fellatio. Secondary lesions in the oral or pharyngeal regions are much less common and may result from indirect causes such as hematogenous spread or autotransmission of organisms from the genital or anal region by contaminated hands or other objects. Any intraoral site may be affected, although the tonsillar region and oropharynx appear to be the most frequent sites of extragenital primary lesions.

The first symptom of an acute gonococcal infection in the mouth may be a burning or itching sensation or a feeling of dryness and heat. This may be followed during the next several days by acute pain as well as increased or decreased salivation. The saliva eventually becomes fetid, and fever and regional lymphadenopathy may or may not develop. The lips may exhibit painful ulcerations, while the gingiva may become erythematous, edematous, painful, and even resemble acute necrotizing ulcerative gingivitis. The tongue may exhibit red denuded areas, as may the soft palate and uvula. Small erythematous lesions resembling herpetic ulcerations or large erythematous lesions may be observed. A diffuse redness of the oropharynx and tonsils may resemble herpangina, and one can only wonder how many of these cases have been mistakenly diagnosed clinically as "strep throat" (Fig 3–10). Many examples of gonococcal pharyngitis or tonsillitis have been so mild that patients have not sought medical treatment, whereas other cases have presented as severe acute infections with associated mucopurulent discharge and regional lymphadenopathy. Despite the presence of *N. gonorrhoeae* organisms in the oropharynx, the disease is seldom believed to be transmitted from this region to a sex partner, and pharyngeal infection is important mainly as a focal source of gonococcemia.

CLINICAL DIAGNOSIS.—Diagnosis of oral or pharyngeal gonorrhea is difficult and requires a high index of suspicion. The clinical differential diagnosis might include streptococcal tonsillitis or pharyngitis, herpetic lesions, infectious mononucleosis, herpangina, erythema multiforme, and scarlet fever.

Secondary gonococcal infections due to hematogenous spread are not commonly reported in the mouth. Disseminated gonococcal infection may result in a characteristic arthritis-dermatitis syndrome that can produce destruction of joints. Other complications of disseminated gonorrhea include sterility, conjunctivitis, erythema multiforme, and serious infections such as endocarditis and meningitis.

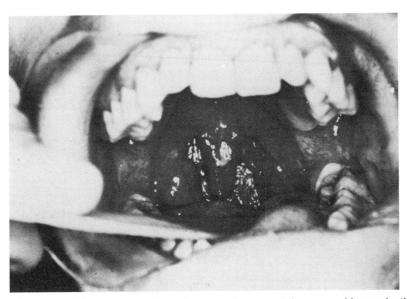

Fig 3–10.—Edematous, erythematous oropharyngeal tissues and hyperplastic tonsillar tissue in primary oropharyngeal gonorrhea. Clinically, this may be mistaken for "strep throat."

DETECTION METHODS.—These include microscopic examination of the exudate from an infected site to detect the presence of gram-negative diplococci intracellularly within leukocytes. A number of *Neisseria* organisms closely resemble each other microscopically, making visual differentiation very difficult. Culturing of the organisms on Thayer-Martin or Transgrow selective media has simplified their differentiation, and positive identification of the organism is made when it is oxidase-positive, ferments only dextrose, and growth is not initiated at 22 to 26 degrees Centigrade. Transport media kits with a carbon dioxide atmosphere are commercially available to enable the dentist to obtain an oral or throat swab and transport the specimen to the laboratory within 3 days. A fluorescent antibody test is also available to assist in the diagnosis of gonorrhea.

TREATMENT.—Penicillin in some form is the treatment of choice, although other antibiotics may be substituted. Occasional cases of penicillinase producing *N. gonorrhoeae* will demonstrate resistance and require therapy with spectinomycin. The dentist and his auxiliary personnel must carefully practice prevention in managing patients with oral gonococcal infections, because transmission to dental personnel or other patients may occur through contaminated instruments or direct contact through a minor hand or finger wound. Patients with or suspected of having active oral/pharyngeal infection should not undergo routine or elective dental therapy. Only urgently required dental treatment should be performed, and the dentist and his assistant should take special precautions to include the wearing of gloves for their own protection. Trauma, such as might be experienced during an extraction, should be minimized during an active oral infection because of the possibility that dental manipulation of an infected area may cause hematogenous spread of the organism or a local gonococcal osteitis of the jaw.

Preventive Measures for Infectious Diseases

It is important for all dental personnel to be thoroughly familiar with reasonable techniques and physical or chemical devices that can afford them some protection against the contraction of disease from the contaminated environment they work in. Most of us are aware of stories in which dental personnel have developed an illness as a result of patient exposure. Unfortunately, instances of anecdotal evidence of disease transmission among our coworkers do not provide direct evidence about transmission of infectious diseases. Consequently, there are a number of our colleagues who believe that we have gone to extremes in recommending infection control measures that are both costly and time-consuming if implemented properly. After all, can we provide irrefutable evidence that dental personnel in significant numbers have contracted serious diseases from their patients, and aren't we dealing with only a remote possibility of a health hazard rather than an actual threat to our way and quality of life? How often we hear comments from dentists who say, "I can't talk to my patients through a mask, and besides, it scares them," or "I don't have any tactile sensation when I wear rubber gloves." Take the example of the dental assistant or dental hygienist who prefers to wear their neat, white, but contaminated uniforms home to their family at the day's end; what possible hazard could there be in this? Statements of this type by skeptics of infection control abound, and proponents have a difficult time convincing them that they do have valid answers or workable solutions for many of their objections.

There is considerable evidence to show now that dental personnel in significant numbers are contracting disease from their patients. The wearing of masks, eye protection, and gloves may indeed be uncomfortable and awkward at first. As to the loss of tactile sensation from wearing gloves, other individuals such as microvascular surgeons or microassembly electronic technicians seem to perform functions requiring tactile sensation and dexterity quite well while wearing surgical rubber gloves. Antibiotics have made us complacent about the management of infection, and even though we may be "shadowboxing" an invisible assailant, we should strive to prevent infection rather than treat it after it has occurred. These remarks often have little impact on the way we conduct our practice until one of us or a close associate develops an incapacitating disease from a patient. How unfortunate this is when the disease was probably preventable if simple precautions had been practiced.

Practical ways to prevent cross-contamination and reduce our exposure level to infectious hazards in the dental environment include the following:

1. Frequently perform a thorough health history and oral examination of each patient. Keep records updated, and note any serious illness or infections that could pose a hazard to you or office personnel.

2. You and your office personnel should periodically have a health physical examination. This is an opportune time to include testing for tuberculosis and HBV.

3. Use a tongue blade and/or gloves to examine suspicious lesions—avoid direct contact.

4. Wear a disposable face mask. These lose their effectiveness when wet and should be changed frequently. The tie-on surgical masks are much more effective than the molded "turtle-shell" mask.

5. Wear disposable gloves. Ideally, these should be worn for all patients, but should particularly be used for examining lesions, performing surgical

procedures, and when cuts or abrasions are present on hands or fingers.

6. Use effective eye protection (unbreakable lenses with side barriers are recommended).

7. Prior to examination or treatment, have patient rinse with an antiseptic mouthwash of your choosing to reduce their oral microbial population.

8. Use high-volume aspiration in conjunction with the rubber dam to minimize splatter and aerosol formation from air/water spray or handpiece. High-volume aspiration is also indicated during use of ultrasonic scaling devices. Polish amalgam restorations, teeth, etc., with a rubber cup instead of a bristle brush. The reader is referred to Chapter 2 for a more thorough discussion of aerosol hazards.

9. Autoclavable handpieces, air/water syringe tips, suction tips, and ultrasonic scaler tips are useful in controlling cross-contamination.

10. Some reduction of microbial contamination can be temporarily achieved by flushing the water lines to the handpiece, air/water syringe, and ultrasonic scaler for at least 2 minutes prior to use after overnight shutdown. Flush lines for at least 4 minutes after a weekend or long period of inactivity. Methods to reduce contamination of unit water lines by use of chemical agents and systems for delivery of sterile water continue to be researched. A few commercial systems are available for unit sterile water delivery.

11. Install antiretraction valves on all unit water lines (if not already in place) to prevent "suck-back." This is easily accomplished and may help to reduce microbial contamination.

12. Use disposable supplies whenever possible.

13. Wear heavy rubber utility gloves to mechanically clean all instruments and burs to remove blood and debris. Then place the items in an ultrasonic cleaner with a fresh detergent solution for optimum cleansing prior to sterilization.

14. Sterilization in the dental office is best achieved by steam autoclaving, unsaturated chemical vapor (chemiclave), or dry heat. Gas sterilization with ethylene oxide is an effective alternative, but too costly and time-consuming for most offices. Sterilizing devices should be monitored by periodic (weekly) biologic spore testing. Chemical processing indicators are useful adjuncts to determine if an instrument pack has been processed, but are not indicators of sterility. Chemical sterilization, such as with 2% alkaline glutaraldehyde, is possible, but time-consuming (up to 10 hours) and corrosive for many instruments. Chemical disinfection may be accomplished by glutaraldehyde, formaldehyde, phenol, chlorine, or iodine-containing compounds. Certain solutions of these agents may be useful in cleaning dental units, chairs, or other environmental surfaces in the dental office.

15. Devote careful attention to office and personal hygiene:

- Use a liquid antiseptic soap: bar soaps may promote bacterial growth.
- Use warm, not hot, water for hand washing.
- Scrub hands lightly with a soft brush and pat gently to dry.
- Do not overtrim fingernails and cuticles.
- Always cover cuts on fingers or hands with a finger cot or glove.

16. Proper humidity and temperature control in the office help allow for efficient functioning of skin and mucous membrane defenses. Optimum humidity is in the 40% to 55% range.

17. Good operatory air flow and turnover of room air will help reduce the number of airborne pathogens. Special filtration systems are available, but are expensive.

18. If in doubt about a patient's infectious disease status, limit your treatment accordingly. You may elect to reappoint the patient or refer them for diagnosis and treatment prior to dental therapy. Observe infection control measures for your protection, particularly in unknown patients requiring emergency dental therapy.

Patients with infectious diseases deserve the same high standards of dental care as any other patient. Infectious disease patients do present certain problems and require special management for the protection of other patients and health care providers. Dental care can be safely delivered to even the high-risk patients such as HBV or tuberculosis patients if certain precautions are taken to prevent cross-contamination and infection of other patients or the dental team. Common sense about treating infectious disease patients dictates that elective dental therapy be postponed during the acute stages of the disease. Ideally, for HBV patients, elective procedures should probably be delayed until the patient is 3 months postjaundice and/ or their liver enzymes have returned to normal or if neutralizing antibody (Anti-HBs) is present. For various reasons, personal or otherwise, not all dental practitioners will elect to treat known high-risk infectious disease patients. While it may be best for these individuals to be treated in the hospital setting where personnel are more familiar with infection control procedures, most dental operatories can be utilized to treat these patients if strict infection control measures are taken. The following dental treatment protocol for high-risk patients such as HBV carriers is suggested:

Before the Patient Arrives

1. If possible, treat patients with acute active disease in a special dental operatory set aside for infectious disease cases such as may be available in

some hospital dental suites. Postpone elective procedures during the acute infectious stages of any disease.

2. Give these patients the last appointment of the day to allow ample time for office cleanup after treatment.

3. Cover bracket tables, adjacent counter tops, handpiece holder, etc. with a disposable surgical drape or a disposable painter's drop cloth.

4. Wrap unit switches, light handles, high-volume evacuation hose and handle, etc., with plastic food wrap held in place by autoclave tape. For very warm or hot surfaces, use aluminum foil instead.

5. Remove from the operatory or cover unnecessary equipment and materials.

During the Appointment

1. Protect the dental team and others by strict adherence to sterile techniques, including the wearing of rubber gloves, gowns, masks, and eye protection.

2. Minimize splatter and aerosol formation during rotary instrument use by use of rubber dam and high-volume evacuation. Where placement of the rubber dam is not possible, use the low-speed handpiece.

3. Use as many disposable items as possible. All instruments should be sterile.

4. If available, use a sterilized autoclavable handpiece. If not available, surface-disinfect the handpiece by chemical wiping and wrap the handpiece in plastic wrap.

5. Operate chair controls through the plastic wrap or use foot controls.

6. Avoid or carefully perform procedures that carry a high risk of skin puncture. Double gloving is recommended.

7. If possible, contaminated instruments should be placed after final usage in a holding solution such as 2% alkaline glutaraldehyde prior to being sterilized.

8. *Do not break the chain of asepsis:* refrain from touching your body, clothing, telephone, dental records, x-rays, etc.

After the Appointment

1. Wrap all instruments loosely in a cloth towel or patient napkin, place them in the sterilizer, and run it through a normal sterilizing cycle. Contaminated instruments are *not* to be mechanically cleaned by dental personnel until after initial sterilization.

2. After initial sterilization, wear heavy rubber utility gloves and clean the instruments very carefully. Clean the instruments in a sink filled with water (rather than scrub the instruments under running water) to prevent

aerosol formation. Ultrasonic cleaning is then recommended for optimum cleaning.

3. Resterilize the instruments in your usual manner.

4. Place all wraps and disposable items in a plastic bag, then double bag and label it "contaminated." Do not seal the bag until after step 9. These bags may be disposed of by incineration. An alternative is to use special heat-resistant plastic bags that are sealed, autoclaved, and then disposed of as normal refuse. Disposal of contaminated trash may be governed by local as well as state regulatory policies, and your local hospital may be able to assist you in disposal of contaminated items.

5. Heat-sensitive, nondisposable items should be decontaminated by immersion in chemical sterilizing solution following the manufacturer's recommendations. If sterilization of these items is required, consult the manufacturer's recommended immersion time to achieve sterilization by use of alkaline glutaraldehyde or other chemical agents.

6. Place contaminated reusable laundry items in a special water-soluble laundry bag and label "contaminated" for benefit of hospital laundry personnel.

7. All contaminated surfaces, including the dental unit, light, switches, sink, uncovered counter tops, etc., should be disinfected. An effective agent for surface disinfection is a commercially available alkaline glutaraldehyde/phenate solution (sporicidin) diluted 1:16, which can be applied by moistened gauze pads. Attempt to keep these environmental surfaces moistened with this solution for at least 15 minutes. Another effective agent for disinfection is an equal mixture of an iodine-containing surgical scrub soap (Betadine) with an equal part of 70% isopropyl alcohol. (Caution: This may stain light-colored vinyls, plastics, and fabrics. Test before using if this is a problem.) Keep environmental surfaces wet with this solution for 30 minutes if possible.

8. Aspirate 2 qt of a dilute sodium hypochlorite solution (one part bleach solution to ten parts water) through the central evacuation and saliva-ejector system.

9. Finally, the cleanup personnel should remove their gloves, gowns, and masks and dispose of these items as instructed in step 4. Protective eyewear should be placed in an alkaline glutaraldehyde solution for 30 minutes. These individuals should then disinfect their face and hands (as should the doctors and other assistants) with a surgical scrub soap.

REFERENCES

Acquired Immune Deficiency Syndrome (AIDS): Precautions for clinical and laboratory staff. *Morbidity Mortality Weekly Rep.* 31:577–579, 1982.

Allen A.M., Taplin D.: "Superficial" fungal and bacterial skin infections, in Diet-

INFECTIOUS AND COMMUNICABLE DISEASES

schy J.M. (ed.): *The Science and Practice of Clinical Medicine.* New York, Grune & Stratton, 1981, vol. 8.

Burket L.W.: *Oral Medicine: Diagnosis and Treatment,* ed. 7. Philadelphia, J.B. Lippincott, Co., 1977.

Burns J.C.: Diagnostic methods for herpes simplex infection: A review. *Oral Surg.* 50:346–349, 1980.

Chue P.W.Y.: Gonorrhea: Its natural history, oral manifestations, diagnosis, treatment, and prevention. *J. Am. Dent. Assoc.* 90:1297–1301, 1975.

Crawford J.J.: New light on the transmissibility of viral hepatitis in dental practice and its control. *J. Am. Dent. Assoc.* 91:829–835, 1975.

Fauchard Academy Poll: Nearly a fourth have contracted illness as a result of practicing dentistry. *Dent. Surv.* 41:29, 1965.

Frick J.R.: Infectious disease hazards. *N.C. Dent. J.* 1:10–13, 1973.

Goldman H.S., Hartman K.S.: Their disease, our unease: Infectious diseases and dental practice. *Ann. Dent.* 38:62–71, 1979.

Immune globulins for protection against viral hepatitis. *Morbidity Mortality Weekly Rep.* 30:423–435, 1981.

Inactivated hepatitis B virus vaccine. *Morbidity Mortality Weekly Rep.* 31:317–328, 1982.

Koppel A.C., Hackleman G.L.: Acute tenosynovitis after puncture wound of a finger by a dental bur. *J. Am. Dent. Assoc.* 76:828, 1968.

McKinney R.V.: Hand, foot, and mouth disease: A viral disease of importance to dentists. *J. Am. Dent. Assoc.* 91:122–126, 1975.

Merchant H.W., Schuster G.S.: Oral gonococcal infection. *J. Am. Dent. Assoc.* 95:807–809, 1977.

Perillo R.P.: The hepatitis viruses: Differential diagnosis, in *Perspectives on Viral Hepatitis.* Abbott Laboratories, 1981.

Perspectives on the control of viral hepatitis, type B. *Morbidity Mortality Weekly Rep.* 25:3–8, 1976.

Ratner J.J., Smith K.O.: Serum antibodies to herpes simplex virus type I during active oral herpes infection. *Infect. Immun.* 27:113–117, 1980.

Rowe N.H., Heine C.S., Kowalski C.J.: Herpetic whitlow: An occupational disease of practicing dentists. *J. Am. Dent. Assoc.* 105:471–473, 1982.

Venereal Disease Fact Sheet. U.S. Department of Health, Education and Welfare, Centers for Disease Control, 1974, vol. 75, p. 8195.

Woodruff G.: Tuberculosis and the dentist. *Aust. Dent. J.* 2:61–66, 1977.

Chapter 4

Mercury: Problems and Control

Harriet S. Goldman, D.D.S., M.P.H.

Historical Background

The utilization of mercury can be traced back to 4,500 B.C. in China, where alchemy was practiced. A Chinese alchemist, Ko Hung, wrote that if one held mercury in his hand, the "evil spirits would be kept away." He practiced what he preached and suffered from severe chronic mercury toxicity. The liquid was also utilized by Greek, Roman, and Arabian physicians of the ancient world. They used it in ointments for the treatment of parasitic diseases, dermatologic conditions, and diseases of the male reproductive organs. In fourteenth century Egypt, Nefertiti used mercury sulfide (cinnabar) for tattooing. The first description of occupational mercury poisoning was in 1473 in a book on goldsmithery. In 1530, it became the treatment of choice for syphilis and was used until 1910 when the arsenicals were shown to be effective. However, later in the 16th century, this cure was found to be worse than the disease, and in certain areas the treatment was discontinued.

For almost a century, up until 1941, the fur and felt hat industry was a major source of occupational mercury poisoning, and the use of mercury was consequently banned. Currently, over 4 million lb of mercury are used annually in the United States, with over 210,000 lb utilized each year in dentistry—about 2.5 lb per dentist. Outside of dentistry, the major uses of mercury are in the electrical preparation of chlorine and caustic soda and in manufacturing electrical apparatus. Other occupations at risk include barometer, monometer, and thermometer makers; fur preservers; tannery workers; taxidermists; insecticide makers; textile printers; and battery makers, among many others.

The Current Problem

The dental profession primarily encounters mercury toxicity from two sources: inhalation of vapors, the primary source, and direct absorption

71

into the tissues from handling mercury-containing compounds. Mercury exists in three forms: the organometallic state (industrial pollution), the inorganic form (mercury salts), and in the elemental or vapor state. It is the latter that presents the hazard in dentistry.

Physical Properties

Mercury is a silver-white liquid that vaporizes at temperatures as low as 10 degrees Farenheit. The vapor is colorless and odorless and volatilizes as the temperature rises. Simple procedures such as the condensation and cutting of amalgam increase mercury volatility. This vapor is readily absorbed by whole blood, is oxidized to the mercuric ion rapidly, and is distributed to the body tissues such as the brain, kidney, heart, lungs, and liver. It does have a predilection for the CNS, and here elimination is very slow. It is excreted primarily through the urinary tract, but to a lesser extent through feces, sweat glands, and growing hair.

Normal mercury blood levels for the United States population with no occupational exposure are from 0 to 5 ng/ml. For dentists, normal levels are 5 to 10 ng/ml. The amount of inorganic mercury that can be tolerated by human beings without damage is not clear, but typical symptoms have been seen at 100 to 200 ng/ml, and frank toxicity has been seen at 400 ng/ml. Normal urinary mercury values for a 24-hour urine sample is 0 to 0.015 mg/L, and according to the National Institute for Occupational Safety and Health (NIOSH), the maximum allowable limit is 0.15 mg/L.

Mercury exposure is of significance because of its cumulative effect on the body. Mercury toxicity in dentistry refers to chronic mercurialism (constant exposure over long periods of time). Consequently, NIOSH has set the threshold limit value (TLV) for the maximum amount of ambient mercury vapor personnel should be exposed to over a 40-hour week at 0.05 mg/m^3 air.

Symptomatology of Chronic Mercurialism

Symptoms of chronic mercurialism include the following:

- Muscular tremors (first observable sign) starting with handwriting and progressing to convulsions.
- Loss of appetite; nausea; diarrhea.
- Nervous excitability; insomnia.
- Headache; mental depression.
- Edema of face and legs.
- Speech disorders.
- Eye affectations.

- Swollen glands and tongue.
- Ulceration of oral mucosa; gingivitis.
- Dark pigmentation of marginal gingiva; gingival recession.
- Metallic taste; foul breath.
- Excess salivation.
- Nephritis.
- Pneumonitis.
- Birth defects in offspring.

Treatment is symptomatic, and poor health as a result of toxicity can last for years. Those affected are given nutritional counseling, told to avoid contact with mercury compounds, and in very severe cases are given drugs to promote urinary excretion. These drugs include dimercaprol (BAL) and penicillamine, but their severe side effects, including renal dysfunction, warrant very close observation of the patient. Indiscriminate use must be avoided.

Extent of the Problem

The health hazards of mercury to the dental profession have been a topic of debate and research in the United States since the 1830s. The dental literature and conference reports have indicated quite a few cases of chronic mercury poisoning. Not all cases have been classical in nature, but there was subtle symptomatology, and consequently a differential diagnosis was difficult. Recent surveys have shown that at least 10% of dental offices in the United States have ambient mercury vapor levels in excess of the TLV of 0.05 mg/m^3 air as recommended by NIOSH. Blood and urinalysis of dentists attending professional meetings have shown that anywhere from 50% to 70% of those tested have mercury levels above normal. These studies have also shown that these increased body mercury levels corresponded with careless practice habits, the number of years in practice, and the amount of mercury used a year. A recent report from the United Kingdom suggested that when compared with control groups, female dentists have a higher abortion rate, greater incidence of premature labor, and an elevated perinatal mortality. No definitive information was provided directly linking mercury to this, but further investigation was suggested. This paper was presented at the International Conference on Mercury Hazards in Dental Practice in 1982. Also presented was the observation that dentists in practice for 20 to 30 years and who had raised body levels of mercury differed psychologically from other dentists in that they had mild psychomotor impairment and a tendency toward stressed behavior. Also demonstrated in this group were a large number of neuropathies, but none were debilitating enough to prevent the individual from practicing.

Sources of Contamination

The greatest potential source of mercury vapor contamination is accidental spillage. Other sources include the following:

- Carpeting in operatories.
- Removing old amalgam restorations.
- Use of ultrasonic compactors.
- Faulty amalgamators.
- Leaking amalgam capsules.
- Capsules with mercury or amalgam residue left in them.
- Expressing excess mercury over the floor.
- Exposure of mercury to heat sources (sterilizers) or warm air.
- Improper storage of scrap amalgam.

Dental Mercury Hygiene

Alert all personnel to the potential hazards of mercury. Knowledge of its toxicity should be a mandatory part of training dental personnel.

Office Monitoring

Good ventilation is the most important step in preventing contamination. Periodic filter replacement in the ventilating system is important, because these filters can act as reservoirs for mercury.

The office should be monitored for mercury vapor once a year and more often if contamination is suspected. If there was a spill, monitoring should be done periodically until a safe threshold is reached. Monitoring can be done by a "sniffing" device, but the vapor level is dependent on the work activity at the time, and therefore only a limited assessment is possible. The ADA recommends the following.

Personal Monitoring

Through various badge monitors, one can evaluate the cumulative mercury exposure over an 8-hour period or longer.

The following are mercury-monitoring devices currently on the dental market and include the sniffers as well as the badge monitors. Please note that none of these have been endorsed, approved, or disapproved by this author or the ADA Council on Dental Materials, Instruments and Equipment:

- Bacharach Instruments: Mercury Vapor Sniffer
- Jerome Instrument Corp.: Gold Film Mercury Vapor Analyzer

- Sunshine Scientific Instrument: Selenium Sulfide Paper Mercury Vapor Detector
- Thermotron: Mercollector-Mercometer
- Automatic Control System Division: Mercury Measurement System
- 3M Co., Occupational Health and Safety
  Products Division: 3M Brand Mercury Vapor Monitor
- Williams Gold Refining Co.: Williams Detector
- Beckman Instruments, Inc.: Mercury Vapor Meter

Dentists should contact their state and city health and labor departments to check if monitoring services are available. The dental societies and dental schools should also be checked. The ADA has a monitoring service available to dental practices.

Biologic Evaluations

Annual urinalysis for mercury content should be performed on all dental personnel. Ideally, one should provide a 24-hour sample or, at the very least, the first specimen voided in the morning. Analyses have been done on hair and nails, and a time-weighted average during several weeks or months can be effectively determined in these tissues.

Office Design

Work areas should minimize mercury contamination. Continuous, seamless sheet flooring that extends up the walls for at least 1 ft is recommended. Carpeting is less desirable from the standpoint of mercury hygiene, because major spills cannot be adequately cleaned up. Cabinet tops should be nonporous and have protective edging or a border to confine spills to the area.

Mercury Storage

1. Mercury should be stored in unbreakable, tightly sealed containers away from any heat.

2. Properly seal all amalgam capsules before amalgamation. There should be no residual amalgam left in reusable capsules, and rubber "O" rings can be used to hold the capsule sections together.

3. Capsules can be checked for leaks by wrapping electrical tape around one section, and if there is leakage during amalgamation, mercury droplets will adhere to the tape.

4. Preproportioned and reusable capsules leak to varying degrees. Therefore, an amalgamator should provide an enclosure for the capsule. The amalgamator should be disassembled periodically to look for and re-

move any accumulated mercury. The arm of the machine should also be checked to ensure a tight fit on the capsule.

5. Because all capsules leak, capsule selection should be based on the tightest fit possible between both halves. With long-term use, leakage occurs in most instances, and therefore the capsules should be replaced periodically.

6. Both types of capsules should be reassembled immediately after dispensing the amalgam, because they represent an important contamination source.

7. Mercury dispenser orifices should be checked for leakage and residual mercury and cleaned after refilling. Some dispensers leak when not in use and should be checked routinely. They should be stored on trays so that leakage, if any, can be retained. The big advantage of the preproportioned capsule is that the chance of accidental mercury spillage is greatly reduced.

Amalgam Handling

1. Use a no-touch technique.

2. Skin exposed to mercury should be cleansed as often as possible.

3. Use the mercury/alloy ration recommended by the manufacturer to eliminate the need for a squeeze cloth.

4. Use high-volume evacuation and water spray when removing old amalgam or finishing new restorations. A wash bottle trap should be used for evacuation whenever possible.

5. Use a face mask to avoid breathing amalgam dust.

6. Do not use ultrasonic compactors to condense amalgam.

7. Select alloys with low creep values.

8. Know the characteristics of the alloy selected.

9. All scrap amalgam should be saved and stored in a tightly closed container preferably containing a sulfide solution such as x-ray or photographic fixer solution. This will prevent vaporization. Glycerine is also relatively effective.

10. After decanting the storing solution, place accumulated scrap in sealed polyethylene bags and give to your scrap dealer.

11. Clean up mercury spills immediately. *Do not use a vacuum cleaner!*
   a. A wash bottle trap or a syringe can recover all visible droplets of mercury.
   b. Strips of adhesive for cleaning up small spills can be utilized.
   c. Decontamination of area with a sulfur-containing compound coats the mercury droplets to prevent vaporization.

There are several mercury spill cleanup kits available commercially. A listing follows, but products mentioned are neither endorsed, approved, or disapproved by this author or the ADA:

* Acton Associates: Hg X
* Bel-Art Products: Mercury Collector; Mercurisorb-Roth Spill Kit
* Dental Control Products, Inc.: Control Mercury Collector
* Futurecraft Corp.: Demerculator
* Markson Sciences, Inc.: Mercury Collector; Mercury Spill Control Kit
* Mercury Vapor Purifier Enterprises: Mercury Vapor Purifier
* Science Related Materials: Hg Vac; SRM Mercury Spill Control Center
* Scientific Services, Inc.: Mercury Spill Cleanup Kit
* VWR Scientific: Mercury Vacupick
* Williams Gold Refining Co.: Williams Protector

Conclusion

Although it is practically impossible to totally eliminate mercury contamination in the dental workplace, adherence to the aforementioned guidelines should minimize mercury toxicity. The key to prevention of contamination is simply reducing the chance that it will escape into the environment.

The adverse effects of mercury poisoning have been investigated by many researchers and are well documented. It behooves the dental profession to be sufficiently informed on both diagnosing and preventing systemic toxicity.

REFERENCES

Battistone G.C., Hefferren J.J., Miller R.A., et al.: Mercury: Its relation to the dentist's health and dental practice characteristics. *J. Am. Dent. Assoc.* 92:1182–1188, 1976.

Bloch P., Shapiro I.M.: Summary of the International Conference on Mercury Hazards in Dental Practice. *J. Am. Dent. Assoc.* 194:989, 1982.

Cooley R.L., Barkmier W.W.: Techniques and devices for recovering mercury and preventing contamination. *Gen. Dentistry* 30:36–41, 1982.

Criteria for a Recommended Standard Occupational Exposure to Inorganic Mercury, HSM 73–11024. U.S. Department of Health, Education and Welfare, National Institute for Occupational Safety and Health.

Friberg L., Vostal J. (eds.): *Mercury in the Environment.* Cleveland, CRC Press, 1972.

Goldman H.S.: Mercury: From alchemy to dentistry. *Dent. Dimensions* July/Sept. 1979.

Goldwater L.F.: *Mercury: A History of Quicksilver*. Baltimore, York Press, 1972.

Harris D., Nicols J.J., Stark R., et al.: The dental working environment and the risks of mercury exposure. *J. Am. Dent. Assoc.* 97:811–815, 1978.

Iyer K., Goodgold J., Eberstein A., et al.: Mercury poisoning in the dentist. *Arch. Neurol.* 33:788–790, 1976.

Mantyla D.G., et al.: Mercury toxicity in the dental office: A neglected problem. *J. Am. Dent. Assoc.* 92:1189, 1976.

Merfield D.P., Taylor A., Gemmel D.M., et al.: Mercury intoxication in a dental surgery following unreported spillage. *Br. Dent. J.* 141:179–186, 1976.

WHO meeting of investigators for international study of normal values for toxic substances. *W.H.O. Occup. Health* 66:39, 1966.

Chapter 5
Potential Hazards of Trace Inhalation Anesthetic Gases

William Greenfield, D.D.S.

DENTISTS AND DENTISTRY have played an extremely important role in all aspects of anesthesia; not only in the discovery of general anesthesia, but also in the early development of the techniques and apparatus used to administer the agents. History has recorded not only these, but also other major contributions made by the dental profession in the field of pain control. Among the techniques of pain control pioneered in dentistry are ultralight levels of anesthesia and conscious sedation utilizing intravenous and inhalation agents, and dentistry can be justifiably proud of its contributions in these most significant areas. It should be noted that in virtually all of these office techniques, as in most every anesthetic administered in the hospital, the use of nitrous oxide is an important part of the anesthetic or sedative regimen, and nitrous oxide is the single most widely used anesthetic/sedative agent.

For the past 10 to 15 years, an increasing number of references in the literature have called attention to a variation in health patterns of individuals clinically exposed to trace amounts of residual inhalation anesthetics. These references have suggested the possibility of a deleterious effect on the health of such personnel. Because an estimated 35% of dentists currently utilize techniques of inhalation sedation and recognizing that office techniques of general anesthesia in which other agents are combined with nitrous oxide are commonly used by oral and maxillofacial surgeons and other dentists, further estimates are that more than 100,000 individuals (dentists, assistants, and other dental office personnel) are chronically exposed to trace concentrations of inhalation anesthetic gases. This is a matter of some concern to a large number of people in dentistry as well as in medicine and those governmental agencies involved in regulation of environmental conditions related to work places. From the first indication that there might be an occupational hazard associated with the use of anesthetic

79

agents, a committee to review and evaluate all current data and to keep the profession informed was established by the American Society of Anesthesiologists (ASA), followed by a similar committee established by the ADA. These committees have taken active roles not only in delineating the potential problem, but also in initiating and supporting appropriate epidemiologic studies in this country.

Historical Review

The earliest epidemiologic study designed to survey occupational health hazards in anesthetists was conducted by Vaisman in Russia in 1967. The study, which included 354 anesthetists, of which 110 were women, was primarily designed to evaluate the working conditions of Russian anesthetists, which Vaisman believed were inadequate. The results of the survey indicated a high incidence of health complaints such as headache, fatigue, and pruritis, which were believed to be associated with inadequate ventilation, poor operating room design, and defective anesthesia equipment. Of particular interest was the unexpected finding that of 31 pregnancies among the 110 female anesthetists, 18 terminated in spontaneous abortion. This same finding of a significantly higher spontaneous abortion rate among female anesthetists was reported in a 1970 Danish study by Askrog and Harvald, with the additional unanticipated finding that wives of male anesthetists also experienced an increased spontaneous abortion rate without having had any direct exposure to the operating room environment. Additional studies conducted in the United States, Great Britain, and Finland produced similar results, with a further indication of a significant increase in congenital abnormalities among children of female anesthetists who worked during pregnancy. In 1973, Corbett and associates published a survey of nurse anesthetists that indicated a much higher incidence of malignancies than in an age-matched control group.

In 1974, an extensive survey of occupational disease among operating room personnel was undertaken by Cohen and others for the ASA Ad Hoc Committee on Effects of Trace Anesthetic Agents on Health of Operating Room Personnel, in cooperation with the National Institute for Occupational Safety and Health (NIOSH). This study, intended to explore the relationship between occupational exposure to anesthetic gases and the incidence of spontaneous abortion, miscarriage, congenital abnormalities, and certain diseases, included individuals in professional societies representing essentially all personnel in the United States potentially exposed to trace gases in the operating room environment. The comparison (control) group included individuals in professional societies working outside of the operating room. Analysis of the results indicated that female anesthesiologists, nurse anesthetists, and operating room nurses and technicians exposed to the operating room during their first trimester of pregnancy, as well as during the preceding year, were subject to a statistically significant increased risk of spontaneous abortion that was 1.3 to 2 times that of the unexposed, nonoperating room personnel. Also, there was evidence for an increased risk of congenital abnormalities among live-born children of exposed females (5.9% in female anesthesiologists compared with 3.0% in unexposed female pediatricians). A statistically significant increase in the incidence of congenital abnormalities was noted also among children of the wives of male operating room-exposed physician anesthetists, possibly suggesting a defect transmitted through the male. The study also indicated an increased risk of cancer and of hepatic and renal diseases in the exposed females. Despite these findings, the authors were careful to point out that the study does not by itself establish a cause-and-effect relationship between reported increased disease rates and specific exposure to waste anesthetic gases in the operating room, because unknown hazards in these locations may have been responsible for the observed results.

With regard to pregnancy, miscarriage, and congenital abnormalities, it should be noted that there are approximately 30,000 anomalous children born in a year, representing 1% to 2.5% of all live births in the United States. Statistics relating cause generally ascribe 20% to genetic influence, 10% to chromosomal damage, and 10% to viruses; 60% are of unknown cause. Many authorities believe the majority of defects occurring in live births represent isolated events unrelated to specific toxic exposure and that toxic reactions generally manifest themselves by causing fetal death rather than malformation unless the exposure is severe enough to cause a 50% mortality. At that point, the surviving fetuses will frequently exhibit abnormalities. The subject is further complicated by the fact that while much teratologic research has been done with animals, the conclusions cannot be freely extrapolated to humans.

Studies in Dental Personnel and Implications to Dentistry

As a separate but distinct part of the 1974 ASA Ad Hoc Committee study outlined above, a preliminary survey of health hazards among dentists was conducted of 4,797 general dental practitioners and 2,642 oral surgeons. The survey indicated a potentially serious occupational health hazard associated with inhalation anesthetic agents, as evidenced by a significant increase (78%) of spontaneous abortion in the spouses of exposed dentists and a significant increase (156%) in liver disease for exposed dentists. Additionally, the study indicated that exposed females had a higher risk of spontaneous abortions, of congenital abnormalities in their children, and of cancer and hepatic and renal disease. No increase in cancer was found in the exposed males, but there was a similar increase in hepatic disease.

Because of the increased interest in the problem and as part of the movement directed to examination of the complex issues relating not only to cause but also to correction of the alleged problem, in February 1976 the ADA named an Ad Hoc Committee on Trace Anesthetics as a Potential Health Hazard in Dentistry. The committee reviewed and evaluated all of the information accumulated to date, and in October 1977 a special-emphasis issue of the *Journal of the American Dental Association* was devoted to the subject of trace inhalation anesthetics in the dental office, including a position paper of the ADA Ad Hoc Committee. The position paper noted that the only epidemiologic study conducted to date with a dental population was deficient in a number of important areas. The major weaknesses included the fact that it was limited in numbers, with less than 7% of the total possible population included (3,000 exposed dentists studied—2,000 oral surgeons and 1,000 general practitioners); no attempt was made to obtain specific information on the most susceptible group, the female, because about 1% of the dentist population is female, and under the protocol of the limited survey, it was not possible to study hygienists, dental assistants, and other involved females; and, most important, no attempt was made to distinguish the specific effects of nitrous oxide alone as a single contaminant (85% of all gases used in dentistry) vs. the other inhalation anesthetic mixtures used. Also, when the data were being compiled, there were not enough exposed general dental practitioners for adequate statistical analysis. Therefore, all exposed general practitioners and oral surgeons were grouped together and measured against all nonexposed general practitioners and oral surgeons. This was believed to be a serious defect in the study. Because of the major deficiencies noted, additional studies oriented specifically to dentistry and delineating specific effects of nitrous oxide as a sole agent were considered essential before any definitive conclusions could be reached. However, despite these reservations, the committee strongly urged that "under the present circumstances every effort should be made to reduce, by presently existing technology, the trace concentration of anesthetic/sedative agents in the dental environment" (Jones and Greenfield). Preliminary to and as part of its recommendation to the profession, the committee emphasized that both general anesthesia and inhalation sedation techniques using the agents in question are considered absolutely essential to the practice of modern pain control in dentistry, and these recommendations were not intended to limit or otherwise curtail the use of inhalation anesthetic and sedative agents in dentistry.

Recognizing and responding to the need for a properly structured large-scale epidemiologic survey of the dental profession and ancillary female personnel with chronic exposure to trace anesthetic gases, a major survey was initiated in 1978, supported by the National Institutes of Health and the ADA. An initial postcard mailing was sent to 138,278 United States dentists to determine inhalation anesthetic or sedative use, with 107,771 responses. From this number, two groups of equal size were subsequently established for questionnaire survey sampling representing approximately 15,000 users of inhalation anesthetics and 15,000 nonusers. A mailing list of approximately 150,000 chairside assistants was developed from a question in the dental form that asked each dentist to supply in the returned questionnaire the names of assisting personnel. The assistants, in turn, were sent a specially prepared questionnaire similar to that the dentists received. From this number, two groups of equal size (approximately 15,000 each) were established representing users and nonusers. By this means, predominantly male (dentists) or female (assistants) control and exposed groups were created. In the exposed groups, two subgroups were created, consisting of those lightly exposed (1 to 8 hours/week) and those heavily exposed (more than 8 hours/week). The specific effects of nitrous oxide alone were clearly distinguished from those of other anesthetic gases. The results of the study, published in another special-emphasis issue of the *Journal of the American Dental Association* in July 1980, seemed to conform, not unexpectedly, to those of previous similar studies in many respects.

The results can be summarized as follows. Spontaneous abortion rates were significantly higher for both wives of exposed dentists and exposed female assistants (1.5 to 2.3 times). The frequency of cancer was not related to anesthetic exposure in either dentists or their assistants. However, health abnormalities clustered under headings of liver, kidney, or neurologic disease were significantly increased in both groups that were heavily exposed to anesthetic gases. In the case of neurologic disease, the increase (1.9 to 2.8 times) was accounted for by nonspecific complaints of numbness, tingling, and muscle weakness rather than specific neurologic diseases. It should be noted that in the lightly exposed groups, the increased incidence of these disease states approached, but did not always achieve, statistical significance. When the effects of nitrous oxide alone were evaluated separately, the results were essentially unchanged. Congenital abnormalities were also found to be significantly more frequent in the children of the female assistants, but here an apparent statistical anomaly was encountered in that this was only true for the lightly exposed group.

In the same issue (July 1980), the ADA Ad Hoc Committee reviewed the study and pointed out that although the total numbers of persons with adverse responses were quite small, the results nonetheless were statistically significant. The same admonition from October 1977 was repeated to the profession, specifically that the dentist should exert every effort to reduce trace concentrations of inhalation anesthetic gases in the dental environment.

Proposals for Regulation

Recommendations for a standard (criteria document) on waste anesthetic gases and vapors were developed by NIOSH in March 1977 for all individuals exposed to inhalation anesthetic agents that escape into locations associated with the administration of or recovery from anesthesia. The recommendations were designed to protect the health of persons during their working lifetimes in locations where exposure to waste anesthetic gases and vapors occur. The criteria document was forwarded to the Occupational Safety and Health Administration for enforcement as written or with modifications. The following criteria from this document are those pertinent to dentists and related to nitrous oxide:

1. Occupational exposure to nitrous oxide, when used as the sole anesthetic agent, shall be controlled so that no worker is exposed to time-weighted average concentrations greater than 25 ppm during anesthetic administration. Available data indicate that with current controlled technology, exposure levels of 50 ppm and less for nitrous oxide are attainable for dental offices.

2. As soon as practicable after promulgation of a standard for occupational exposure to waste anesthetic gases, anesthetic delivery systems shall be equipped for scavenging.

3. Medical surveillance shall be made available to all employees subject to occupational exposure to waste anesthetic gases.

Comprehensive preplacement medical and occupational histories shall be obtained and maintained in each employee's medical records, with special attention given to the outcome of pregnancies of the employee or spouse, and to hepatic, renal, and hematopoietic systems which may be affected by agents used as anesthetic gases. This information should be updated at least yearly and at any other time considered appropriate by the responsible physician.

The preplacement and annual physical examination of employees exposed to anesthetic gases are recommended and, when performed, the results shall be maintained in the employee's permanent records.

Employees shall be advised of potential undesirable effects of exposure to waste anesthetic gases such as spontaneous abortions, congenital anomalies in their children, and effects on the liver and kidneys.

Any abnormal outcome of the pregnancies of the employees or of the spouses of employees exposed to anesthetic gases shall be documented as part of the employee's medical records, and records shall be maintained for the period of employment plus 20 years. This medical information shall be available to the designated medical representatives of the Secretary of Health, Education and Welfare, of the Secretary of Labor, of the employees or former employees, and of the employer.

4. Containers of gaseous and volatile anesthetic agents shall carry labels.

5. On assignment and at least annually thereafter, each worker shall be informed of the possible health effects of exposure to waste anesthetic gases. This information shall emphasize the potential risks to workers of reproductive age and to their unborn children. Each worker shall be instructed as to the availability of such information, which shall be kept on file and shall be accessible to the worker in each place of employment where a potential exposure to waste anesthetic gases exists.

6. A monitoring program shall be supervised by an eligible individual with sampling and monitoring techniques or by a professional industrial hygienist. The agent to be monitored and the method chosen will depend on the frequency of the agent's use, availability of sampling and analysis instrumentation, and on whether the facility chooses to initiate its own monitoring program or take advantage of commercial service.

7. Records of all collected air samples shall be maintained including date of sample, sampling methods, sampling location, analytical methods, and measured concentrations. If waste anesthetic gas levels are found above the environmental limits prescribed, corrective actions shall be taken and recorded. Results of environmental measurements shall be made available to exposed employees on request. Air sampling results and results of leak tests shall be maintained for at least 20 years. Medical records shall be kept for the duration of employment plus 20 years after an employee's termination of employment or termination of work of a self-employed person.

The following definitions apply to the above concepts:

Time Weighted Average (TWA) – This type of sampling is frequently employed for checking air contamination. A TWA sample is obtained by pumping ambient air continuously into an inert bag at constant low flow rates; the bag concentration then represents average exposure. The integrated output of an infrared analyzer will also provide a TWA.

ppm – Low concentrations of gas are expressed on a volume/volume basis as parts per million (ppm). Thus, 100% of a gas equals 1,000,000 ppm, 1% of a gas equals 10,000 ppm. It should be noted that in operating rooms where no attempt has been made to reduce leakage or to scavenge waste gases, trace gas levels can approximate 500 ppm for nitrous oxide, and in dental offices, levels can be two or three times this amount.

Recommendations to the Dentist

1. Every dental office or facility in which inhalation anesthetic/sedative gases are used should have an effective program of scavenging and monitoring. Devices in these categories that combine effectiveness with practicality are currently available. Guidelines for scavenging equipment and for monitoring devices have been promulgated by the ADA Council on Dental Materials, Instruments and Equipment.*

---

*From Expansion of the acceptance program: Nitrous oxide scavenging equipment and nitrous oxide trace gas monitoring equipment. ADA Council on Dental Materials, Instruments and Equipment. *J. Am. Dent. Assoc.* 95:791–792, 1977. Used by permission.

2. Monitor office for nitrous oxide at the time nitrous oxide equipment is installed and at 4-month intervals thereafter. Attempt to maintain less than 50 ppm nitrous oxide in the dental office.

3. Check nitrous oxide machine, lines, hoses, and mask for leakage.

4. Maintain adequate ventilation. The maximum circulation and venting to the outside should be achieved with a minimum of recirculation. Well-functioning air conditioning and heating units that provide fresh air dilution will aid in the dispersal of the gas from the operatory and decrease the trace concentrations about the dentist and dental assistants.

5. Check to make sure air ventilation systems are functioning properly.

6. Use high-speed evacuation systems vented to the outside.

7. Minimize talking with the patient and, if possible, use a rubber dam.

8. Use an air-sweep fan that blows across the patient and increases mixing of air with nitrous oxide adjacent to operators.

9. Modify the air conditioning system to be of the nonrecirculating type.

10. Exhaust waste gas away from windows, ventilators, air conditioning inlets, or other areas that might provide entrance back into the office. A roof exhaust, for example, might solve the problem.

11. Check the fit of the face mask.

12. Maintain and service equipment regularly.

13. Employ a method of nitrous oxide/oxygen administration that does not allow admixture of room air. Such a technique requires increased nitrous oxide concentrations and flow rates from the machine to reach the desired alveolar air concentration.†

Discussion

The results of the above epidemiologic studies and others have been variously interpreted: some reviewers believe there is convincing evidence of occupational health risk, while others believe these data are inconsistent and that a firm cause-and-effect relationship between chronic exposure to trace levels of anesthetic gases and disease entities in operating room personnel does not exist. These latter reviewers point out that all of the studies are retrospective epidemiologic surveys and suffer from potential errors inherent in such studies, including possible responder bias, inaccurate recall, and the possible impact of the unknown results in nonresponders. Still, the results of the most recent large-scale dental study are largely consistent with those reported from previous surveys and support the gen-

---

†From ADA Council on Dental Materials, Instruments and Equipment: *Dentist's Desk Reference: Materials, Instruments and Equipment*. Chicago, American Dental Association, 1981, p. 25. Used by permission.

eral conclusion that anesthetic contamination appears to be a potential health hazard for exposed workers. This conclusion is particularly strengthened by the apparent dose-response relationship that was observed for spontaneous abortion as well as for kidney, liver, and neurologic diseases.

To point up the controversy, a study recently conducted at the ADA Health Foundation Research Institute and supported in part by NIOSH showed that continuous nitrous oxide exposure at levels far above those found in dental offices failed to produce kidney or liver damage in laboratory rats, leading researchers to rethink the implications of nitrous oxide as an occupational hazard in dentistry. In this study, both male and nonpregnant female rats were exposed to 1% to 2% nitrous oxide continously for up to 84 days. During the same time, control rats were exposed to normal room air. At the end of the exposure period, which was as much as 200 times higher than that to which dental workers are exposed (which is always intermittent), the rats were examined by standard biochemical techniques that indicate liver and kidney function. The results revealed no significant adverse effects on either male or female rat livers and kidneys. Researchers noted that tissue examination concurred with the biochemical results.

Regardless of the position one takes regarding the value of the data related to potential health hazards of waste anesthetic gases, one of the questions that often comes up concerns information that should be given to employees that work in areas where they will be exposed to such gases. The ASA Ad Hoc Committee has addressed this question and in an informational brochure to its members offers the following suggested notification to potentially exposed employees:

PERSONNEL NOTICE*

Notice to Employees on the Possible Potential Health Hazards Associated with Occupational Exposure to Anesthetics

Our concern about your health and the quality of our environment requires that we periodically bring to your attention the suspected occupational health hazards associated with working in anesthetizing locations such as the operating room.

Epidemiologic surveys suggest that there may be increased incidences of some diseases, particularly those associated with the reproductive process, in operating room employees.

While chronic occupational exposure to trace concentrations of anesthetic gases is a suspected cause of these disease entities, the evidence is equivocal. Thus, conclusive proof of cause is presently not available.

---

*From ASA Waste Anesthetic Gases in Operating Room Air: A Suggested Program to Reduce Personnel Exposure. Chicago, American Society of Anesthesiologists, p. 19. Used by permission.

Indeed, other factors such as the stress of working in the operating room have also been proposed as causes of these health hazards.

Fortunately, anesthetic exposure can be reduced substantially. A comprehensive protection program is in effect in all of our surgical and obstetric operating rooms: equipment maintenance has reduced leakage to a minimum; excess anesthetic circuit gases are captured and vented at a point where no personnel exposure occurs; and the operating room air is monitored to document that the trace gas control program is effective and that low levels really are being maintained.

A question frequently raised is whether women who are pregnant or who are contemplating pregnancy should work in the operating room. A definite answer cannot be given, and the data are not strong enough to remove categorically all such women from the operating rooms. With the above factors in mind, we have attempted to make our operating suites as safe as possible by our concerted efforts to hold anesthetic exposure to a minimum. However, no "safe" exposure level below which we can be sure that adverse effects will not occur has yet been identified. You must decide whether to accept the potential risks of working in anesthetizing areas. Should you have any questions or concerns, we urge that you consult your obstetrician or a knowledgeable anesthesia department member.

Whether pregnant or not, if you prefer not to have any exposure to trace gases, then you may request to work elsewhere in the hospital. The staff in the Anesthesia, Surgical, Nursing, and Housekeeping Departments will make every effort to accommodate the wishes of concerned persons.

To show that you have received and understand this notice, please sign below and return it to us.

Thank you for your cooperation.

I have read and understand this notice.

_____

Name

_____

Date

Summary

An increasing series of retrospective epidemiologic surveys appears to indicate that chronic exposure to anesthetic gases can be harmful. There is considerable controversy regarding the establishment of a firm cause-and-effect relationship, and there is no precise indication of the concentration level at which deleterious effects would start to take place. Additional prospective studies of humans, as well as additional animal studies, are needed to further define the extent of the potential problem.

However, despite the controversial nature of the issue, it is recommended that the dentist exert every effort to reduce trace concentrations of inhalation anesthetic gases in the dental environment. Compliance with this recommendation presupposes an effective program of scavenging and monitoring. It is important to note also that any potential problems indicated relate strictly to dental personnel with chronic exposure to trace anesthetic gases and do not in any way involve patients, whose exposure to anesthetic gases is of a therapeutic and relatively brief nature.

It must be emphasized also that this is not to be construed as a recommendation to limit the use of inhalation anesthetic or sedative agents or techniques. Inhalation sedation and general anesthesia using nitrous oxide and other agents are essential components of modern control of pain in dentistry, as they are in medicine, and there is no intent in these recommendations to curtail the use of these agents or techniques. Their current use and future development is actively encouraged, together with the continued development of more effective monitoring and scavenging techniques.

REFERENCES

ADA Council on Dental Materials, Instruments and Equipment: *Dentists's Desk Reference: Materials, Instruments and Equipment.* Chicago, American Dental Association, 1981, p. 25.

Archer W.II.: The history of anesthesia, in Archer W.H. (ed.): *Oral Surgery Directory of the World,* ed. 4. Ann Arbor, Mich., Edward Bros., 1971, p. 385.

ASA Waste Anesthetic Gases in Operating Room Air: A Suggested Program to Reduce Personnel Exposure. Chicago, American Society of Anesthesiologists, p. 19.

Askrog V., Harvald B.: Teratogenic effects of inhalation anesthetics. *Nord. Med.* 83:498–500, 1970.

Cohen E.N.: *Anesthetic Exposure in the Workplace.* Littleton, Mass., Wright, John, PSG, Inc., 1980.

Cohen E.N., Bellville, J.W., Brown B.W.: Anesthesia, pregnancy, and miscarriage: A study of operating room nurses and anesthetists. *Anesthesiology* 35:343–347, 1971.

Cohen E.N., Brahm B.W., Bruce D.L., et al.: Occupational disease among operating room personnel: A national study. *Anesthesiology* 41:321–340, 1974.

Cohen E.N., Brown B.W., Bruce D.L., et al.: A survey of anesthetic health hazards among dentists. *J. Am. Dent. Assoc.* 90:1291–1296, 1975.

Cohen E.N., Gift H.C., Brown B.W., et al.: Occupational disease in dentistry and chronic exposure to trace anesthetic gases. *J. Am. Dent. Assoc.* 101:21–31, 1980.

Corbett T.H., Cornell R.G., Lieding K., et al.: Incidence of cancer among Michigan nurse-anesthetists. *Anesthesiology* 38:260–263, 1973.

Criteria for a Recommended Standard . . .Occupational Exposure to Waste Anesthetic Gases and Vapors. U.S. Department of Health, Education and Welfare, National Institute for Occupational Safety and Health, 1977.

Expansion of the acceptance program: Nitrous oxide scavenging equipment and nitrous oxide trace gas monitoring equipment. ADA Council on Dental Materials, Instruments and Equipment. *J. Am. Dent. Assoc.* 95:791–792, 1977.

Greenfield W.: Commentary: Potential hazards of chronic exposure to trace anesthetic gases: Implications for dentistry. *J. Am. Dent. Assoc.* 101:158–159, 1980.

Jastak J.T., Greenfield W.: Trace contamination of anesthetic gases: A brief review. *J. Am. Dent. Assoc.* 95:758–762, 1977.

Jones T.W., Greenfield W.: Position paper of the ADA Ad Hoc Committee on Trace Anesthetics as a Potential Health Hazard in Dentistry. *J. Am. Dent. Assoc.* 95:751–756, 1977.

Knill-Jones R.P., Moir D.D., Rodriguez L.V., et al.: Anesthetic practice and pregnancy: Controlled survey of women anesthetics in the United Kingdom. *Lancet* 2:1326–1328, 1972.

News item. *ADA News,* April 11, 1983, p. 2.

Rosenberg P.H., Kirves A.: Miscarriages among operating room staff. *Acta Anaesthesiol. Scand.* 53(suppl.):37–42, 1943.

Smith B.E.: Teratology in anesthesia. *Clin. Obstet. Gynecol.* 17:145, 1974.

Vaisman A.I.: Working conditions in surgery and their effect on health of anesthesiologists. *Eksp. Khir. Anestheziol.* 3:44–49, 1967.

Chapter 6

Physical, Chemical, and Thermal Injuries*

Robert L. Cooley, D.M.D., M.S.

PHYSICAL, CHEMICAL, AND THERMAL agents encompass a wide range of potential health risks. An attempt will be made in this chapter to discuss the most obvious of these hazards, but some that others consider important may be omitted. The dangers of these agents will be presented as occupational hazards to those employed in the dental office, but they may also pose great hazards to the patients. This should be taken into consideration whenever patients are present. Many of these hazards can be minimized by using common sense and by observing some simple precautions.

Physical Hazards

Physical agents are usually thought of as objects that can be seen or felt. However, the National Institute for Occupational Safety and Health (NIOSH) defines a physical agent as an entity without substance or with minimal matter, such as radiation, atmospheric variations, noise, and vibration. Although without substance, these agents have a potentially adverse effect on the exposed individual. Ionizing radiation and noise will be considered in other chapters. Physical hazards to be discussed in this section include eye injuries, ultraviolet radiation, visible light radiation, puncture wounds from burs and instruments, radiofrequency and microwave radiation, and asbestos.

Eye Injuries

The dental environment presents a threat to the vision of both dental personnel and patients. A number of instruments routinely used by the dentist can cause eye injuries. One in particular, the air-turbine handpiece,

---

*The views and opinions expressed herein are those of the author and do not necessarily reflect the views of the United States Air Force or the Department of Defense.

has an awesome ability to produce eye injuries. Its high rotational speed can turn tooth, amalgam particles, or a dental bur into high-speed projectiles that may cause extensive damage to ocular tissues. Most practitioners have witnessed these projectiles occasionally fly across the operatory, striking walls and equipment with considerable force. Calculus may also become a projectile when scaling procedures are performed. The impact force of calculus does not pose as great a danger as do the microorganisms it contains. These microbes, along with the physical injury, may initiate an eye infection that is difficult to control. Chemicals such as the acids and bases that are used routinely in some dental offices present a special hazard to the eyes. Dental instruments, many of which are sharp, are an ever-present cause of penetrating wounds. The dental lathe is also a particularly dangerous device, because it can turn castings and dental materials into high-speed projectiles that strike with great force.

A number of eye injuries that have occurred in the dental setting have been reported in the literature. It is important to be aware of these injuries so that steps can be taken to prevent their recurrence. Some of these mishaps are briefly described below:

- An explorer being passed over a patient's face was dropped, penetrating his eye and resulting in loss of vision.
- A suture needle penetrated a patient's eye during a surgical procedure, resulting in a massive infection and loss of the eye.
- An excavator was pulled from the bracket table on a gauze pad and penetrated a patient's eye. While vision impairment did occur, total vision was not lost.
- During a chairside denture adjustment, a piece of denture material flew into the patient's eye and caused a corneal abrasion.
- An anesthetic cartridge burst, sending glass into the patient's eye and resulting in a corneal abrasion.
- A crown of a tooth fractured during extraction and struck the dentist's eye with enough force to cause internal bleeding.
- A number of dentists and assistants have received eye injuries from high-speed projectiles. Most of these have been a result of the air-turbine handpiece.

Emergency Treatment

FOREIGN BODIES.—A foreign body should be removed immediately, because it could result in a corneal abrasion (the removal of a portion of the epithelium of the cornea see Figs 6–1 and 6–2). If it can be seen, the foreign body should be removed with a cotton tip applicator or by irrigation

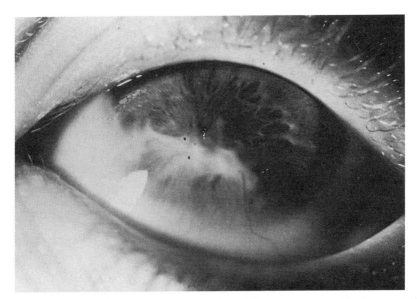

Fig 6–1.—Corneal scar across the center of the eye as a result of a corneal abrasion. A foreign body or high-speed projectile can cause this type of injury. (From Cooley R.L., Barkmeir W.W.: Prevention of eye injuries in the dental office. *Quintessence International* 9:953, 1981. Used by permission.)

with tap water. If it cannot be located or removed, an ophthalmologist should be consulted.

CHEMICAL INJURIES.—These are the most urgent of ocular injuries (Fig 6–3). Irrigation with tap water should begin immediately and continue for 5 to 10 minutes. An ophthalmologist should be consulted immediately for specialized care.

PENETRATING WOUNDS.—These may be caused by an instrument or high-speed projectile (Fig 6–4). Such wounds should be treated by covering them with a firm dressing. This can be accomplished by closing the eye, placing a 2 × 2-in. gauze pad over it, then running two strips of tape from the forehead to the cheek. Immediate consultation with an ophthalmologist is necessary for specialized treatment.

Preventive Techniques

- Never pass instruments or chemicals over the patient's face.
- Perform chairside denture adjustments at a safe distance from the patient.

- Educate the entire dental staff regarding the serious nature of eye injuries.
- Safety glasses should be worn by the dental staff and the patient.

The dentist, assistant, hygienist, and laboratory technician should wear safety glasses when operating rotary instruments or scaling teeth; safety glasses should be provided for the patient as well. Prescription lenses will also protect against high-speed projectiles and instruments. Inexpensive safety glasses, such as the plastic type, can be obtained from several sources. Safety glasses that are fashionable and comfortable (and therefore more likely to be used routinely) can be obtained from local optical shops.

Ultraviolet Radiation

All personnel should be aware of the risks associated with ultraviolet exposure and the sources of this radiation. Dental personnel may be exposed to ultraviolet radiation from several sources and not be aware of this hazard, because it is silent and invisible.

Sources of ultraviolet radiation include ultraviolet generators for curing restorative resins and pit and fissure sealants, ultraviolet plaque lights, il-

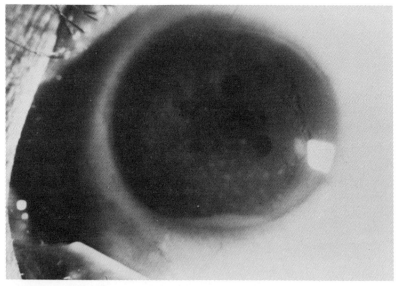

Fig 6–2.—Irregularly shaped pupil with pus collecting in lower part of the eye as a result of traumatic injury. Foreign bodies, corneal abrasions, or traumatic injuries may lead to this type of inflammation of the iris and ciliary body. (From Cooley R.L., Barkmeir W.W.: Prevention of eye injuries in the dental office. *Quintessence International* 9:953, 1981. Used by permission.)

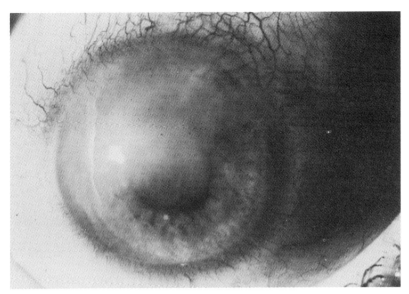

Fig 6–3.—Frosty or misty appearance of eye as a result of chemical injury. Chemical injuries may be caused by acids or alkalies. (From Cooley R.L., Barkmeir W.W.: Prevention of eye injuries in the dental office. *Quintessence International* 9:953, 1981. Used by permission.)

lumination for intraoral photography, and molten metal used for casting.

The hazards that ultraviolet radiation pose to the individual depend on the following factors: (1) intensity of the radiation, (2) time exposed, (3) distance from the source, (4) individual sensitivity, and (5) sensitizing agents or conditions. The potential health risks include (1) conjunctivitis, photokeratitis, and other eye irritations; (2) erythema of skin or mucous membranes; (3) precipitation of herpes simplex lesions, and (4) possible alteration of cells and viruses that transforms the virus to a more oncogenic type and makes the cells more susceptible to this new virus form.

Agents and conditions that may cause hypersensitivity to ultraviolet radiation include plants (figs, limes, parsnips, and pink-rot celery), drugs (tetracycline and 8-methoxypsoralen), and medical conditions (lupus erythematosus, xeroderma pigmentosum, and erythropoietic porphyria). Photosensitizing chemicals called furocoumarins and psoralens in the plants are believed to cause hypersensitivity to ultraviolet radiation.

Personal Protection

With the advent of the visible light-cured resins and improved self-curing resins, the use of ultraviolet-cured resins should be decreasing. Thus,

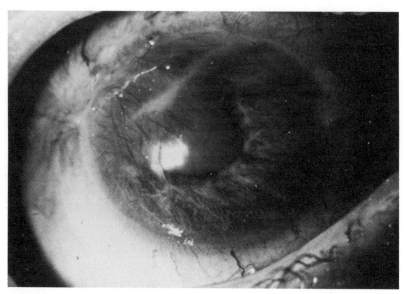

Fig 6–4.—Corneal-sclera laceration, a penetrating wound requiring immediate treatment. Penetrating wounds may be caused by high-speed projectiles or instruments and result in the loss of aqueous humor from the anterior chamber. (From Cooley R.L., Barkmeir W.W.: Prevention of eye injuries in the dental office. *Quintessence International* 9:953, 1981. Used by permission.)

exposure should also be decreasing. However, if the ultraviolet-cured resins are being used routinely and frequently, the following protective measures are recommended:

1. Protective glasses to filter out the ultraviolet radiation.
2. Use of rubber dam to protect the patient's tissues.
3. Proper shielding of the ultraviolet generator to prevent stray exposure.
4. Use of ultraviolet light for the shortest possible time to accomplish procedure.
5. Application of ultraviolet light only to area being treated.
6. Strong consideration of use of visible light-cured resins.

Ultraviolet Radiation From Molten Metals

One study indicates that molten metals heated for casting procedures emit both ultraviolet and infrared radiation. Both may cause injury to the eyes. Laboratory technicians reported that casting and soldering caused eye strain, spots in visual field, headaches, and loss of visual acuity. Protective glasses with green absorptive lenses were recommended. Such lenses filter out both ultraviolet and infrared radiation and are made by Bausch & Lomb under the name of Ray-Ban.®

Visible Light Radiation

Visible light-cured resins are available from a number of manufacturers and offer several advantages over the ultraviolet-cured resins. These resins are cured by an intense visible light from a halogen lamp. Some dentists and assistants have reported "afterimages" from looking at this intense visible light. At present, little is known about the effects of this radiation on human eyes. Both the Council on Dental Materials and the Bureau of Radiological Health are evaluating these devices and their effects on vision. A number of animal studies evaluating the effects of visible light on the optic system have been accomplished. Some of the results of these studies are as follows:

1. Retinal damage from long-term exposure or frequent short-term exposure to intense light sources.

2. Yellowing of the lens of the eye.

3. Retinal damage after a 1-hour exposure to 40-W fluorescent lamps and irreversible retinal damage after 1-week exposure. The 1-week exposure resulted in complete destruction of the photoreceptor cells.

4. Retinal damage from the projection of an indirect ophthalmoscope on the retina for 1 hour. A 5-month follow-up did show evidence of regeneration and repair of the photoreceptor cells.

Factors that may affect retinal damage are length of exposure, brightness of the light, pigmentation of the fundus (of eye), blood pressure, and genetic factors.

Until more is known about the effects of intense visible light, the following recommendations are offered:

1. Warn everyone concerned *not* to stare or look directly at the light source. This includes the dentist, assistant, and patients.

2. Protective glasses should be worn if the visible light source is used frequently or for long periods. One recommendation has been the UV 400 Orcolite lens (Orcolite Corp. Azusa, Calif.).

3. Use a light probe which has a cowl around the tip to prevent stray or reflected light. The Elipar light probe (available from P.O. Box 111, Norristown, Pa.) has such a cowl, and it acts as a shield to limit stray or reflected light.

Puncture Wounds From Burs and Instruments

Scratches and puncture wounds from contact with burs and instruments are possibly the most common of dental injuries. Burs left in handpieces can cause serious injury by piercing soft tissue and then breaking off. Surgical removal may be necessary to remove the fractured segment. The following cases are presented to illustrate the serious nature of this problem:

- A bur came in contact with the operator's finger and fractured. Surgery was required to remove the fractured segment.
- A bur was left in the handpiece of a cart-type unit. The dentist's hip came in contact with the bur, and it fractured. Surgery was required to remove the broken bur from the hip.
- A contaminated bur caused a puncture wound of the finger, resulting in an infection of that finger.
- A bur fractured during the operation of the air turbine, creating a high-speed projectile. The fractured portion of the bur pierced the operator's forehead and had to be surgically removed.

Precautions for Burs

1. Remove burs from handpieces when their use is completed.
2. Never use a bur that has been bent or straightened.
3. Place a cotton roll over burs that have to be left in the handpiece.
4. Do not use the bracket table top or other surface to insert burs in the handpiece, because this may result in a bent bur or an accident that creates a puncture wound.
5. Use only the manufacturer's recommended bur changer to remove and insert burs. Other devices may damage the bur or allow an injury to the fingers.

Precautions for Instruments

1. Sharp instruments in a sterilization pack should have a cotton roll on the sharp end to prevent perforation.
2. Keep instruments on the bracket table in order and do not allow them to become entangled in gauze or other materials.
3. Keep instruments in a cabinet or in a pack when not in use.
4. Pass the blunt end of instruments to the receiver.
5. Use hemostat to put blades on the scalpel handle. Discard blades in the original container or a wrapping to prevent injury to the housekeeping personnel.

Treatment for an Injury

1. Thoroughly wash the injured area with soap and water or with an iodine scrub.
2. Treat the wound with an antiseptic.

3. Check both the bur or instrument and the wound to determine if any fractured segments are present.

4. Obtain antitetanus injection if immunizations are not current.

5. Consult a physician if a foreign body is in the wound, if pain persists, or if an infection occurs.

Radiofrequency and Microwave Radiation

Occupational hazards from radiofrequency and microwave radiation are minimal in dentistry. There appear to be only two items of concern in this category: pacemaker interference and diathermy units.

Pacemaker Interference

Certain types of unshielded pacemakers (the older types) are subject to interference from electromagnetic radiation. This radiation could be emitted by radar, microwave ovens, diathermy units, and also from some dental equipment. Dental equipment that should be used with *caution* around cardiac pacemakers include electrosurgical units, ultrasonic scalers, induction casting machines, diathermy units, and electric toothbrushes.

Both the patient and dental staff who have pacemakers should be aware of the problems associated with electromagnetic interference. The following recommendations are offered to prevent pacemaker arrhythmia:

1. Persons with cardiac pacemakers should avoid dental devices that emit electromagnetic interference.

2. Know or try to determine the type of pacemaker and its ability to reject interference.

3. If in doubt, consult the cardiologist of the concerned individual.

Diathermy Units

Diathermy units are microwave generators used to apply penetrating heat to selected areas of the body. In dentistry, they may be used after extractions and oral surgery procedures, myofacial pain dysfunction, and for traumatic injuries. Hazards of use include burns, tissue necrosis, and electric shock. Suggested precautions are to minimize exposure, carefully place the emitting device, and give attention to output settings. Both the hazards and precautions apply more to the patient than the operator. The operator is not likely to experience burns or tissue necrosis unless there is misuse of the unit or ignorance of the dangers.

Asbestos

Asbestos is a general term that may be applied to any one of a number of minerals that can be crushed into fibers. Asbestos is principally used in dentistry for lining material for casting rings and crucibles, as a binder in periodontal dressings, and for soldering investments.

Asbestos presents serious hazards to health. These include cancer of the lung, pleural cavity, and gastrointestinal tract and pulmonary asbestosis and fibrosis. The following precautions are suggested:

1. Avoid use of ring and crucible lining material that is made of asbestos. Asbestos substitutes are available that are made of spun fired clay such as Kaoliner.®

2. Avoid the use of periodontal dressings and soldering investments that contain asbestos.

3. If asbestos-type materials must be used, the following recommendations are offered:

    a. Wear a face mask and gloves. Wash hands thoroughly after using.

    b. Cut the liner material (do not tear).

    c. Wet asbestos liner material before using to reduce the airborne fibers.

    d. Prohibit smoking, drinking, or eating in the area where asbestos is used.

    e. Work on asbestos only under local exhaust system.

    f. Inform all personnel of the hazards.

Thermal Hazards

There are many opportunities for thermal injuries in the dental environment. Some of these are obvious and merely require a common sense approach and attention to handling and placement. Thermal injuries may be produced from two general sources: (1) flammable liquids and (2) heated instruments, materials, and devices such as compound sticks, autoclaves, chemical vapor, and glass bead sterilizers, gutta-percha points, heat-producing resins, compound heaters, gas burners, alcohol torches, and lamps in dental lights.

Precautions for Heated Instruments

Heated instruments and devices should be handled carefully and are *not* to be passed over or near people. Instruments recently removed from an autoclave should be so labled or placed where another person will not pick them up. Glass bead sterilizers, autoclaves, chemical vapor sterilizers, and alcohol torches should be placed where they will not be tipped over or pulled off a table onto another person. Lamps in dental lights get extremely hot and should not be touched. If these lamps have to be changed, then they should be allowed to cool, or a thick towel may be used as an insulator during removal. There are some cases where these lamps (and their shields) have fallen on patients and caused burns to the individual trying to recover the hot lamp. Therefore, the lamp should be checked occasionally to ensure that it is securely in the socket.

Precautions for Flammable Liquids

Many volatile, highly flammable liquids are used in dentistry. If not stored properly or if used carelessly near flames, a fire or explosion could occur and result in serious burns. Liquids posing this hazard include the following:

1. Ethyl ether
2. Ethyl alcohol
3. Methyl alcohol
4. Isopropyl alcohol
5. Acrylic monomers
6. Acetone
7. Benzene
8. Toluene
9. Methyl ethyl ketone
10. Vapor from chemical sterilizers

The following precautions are suggested:

1. Do not use these liquids near an open flame.
2. Do not store them near an open flame or heat source.
3. Keep these liquids in the original container or a correctly labeled container.
4. Use special storage cabinets for flammable liquids and materials.
5. Fire extinguishers should be available in areas where these liquids are used. The A-B-C type fire extinguisher has been recommended.
6. If large amounts of these liquids are stocked, more stringent storage procedures should be followed, including physical separation from the work areas. Consultation with the local fire marshal may also be prudent.

Fumes From Chemical Vapor Sterilizers

Solutions for chemical vapor sterilizers may contain ethyl alcohol, isopropyl alcohol, methyl alcohol, acetone, and methyl ethyl ketone. This mixture is flammable, and particularly so when it comes out of the sterilizer in vapor form. When the door of the sterilizer is opened, a plume of this chemical vapor comes out and rises toward the ceiling. This chemical vapor has been demonstrated to ignite with an open flame. Therefore, the door of a chemical sterilizer should not be opened when a flame is present. Also, the sterilizer should have a spark-proof power switch, because a flash fire may occur if the door is opened while at the same time the switch is turned off. Some sterilizers have been recalled by the FDA to correct this problem.

Ethylene Oxide Sterilizers

The use of ethylene oxide as a sterilant in dental offices is becoming more common. Dangerous quantities of ethylene oxide gas can be released from sterilizers during their routine use. To minimize exposure to this highly toxic substance, a number of precautions should be taken. Sterilizers should be exhausted to a safe outdoor location and purged with a sufficient volume of air before being opened. Interlocks should be provided to prevent opening of the sterilizers while they are being used. Periodic checks should be made of the equipment to detect leaking and any other malfunctioning parts. Sterilized items may retain ethylene oxide, and skin irritation can result from contact with these items. Protective gloves and forceps should be used whenever possible to remove items from sterilizers. Since ethylene oxide gas is extremely flammable, it should be used only in areas in which all sources of ignition are strictly controlled. These areas must also be well ventilated to insure dissipation of any liberated gas.

Chemical Hazards

This section will identify chemicals that present an occupational risk as well as those metals in dental alloys that may be hazardous. Except for the first subject, these chemicals will be discussed in the following groups: acids, alkalies, organic compounds, gypsum products, and x-ray chemicals.

Chemicals Causing Dermatoses

Occupational dermatosis has been defined as an abnormality of the skin that is caused by the occupational environment. Dermatoses is a term designating a group of skin disorders that may include (1) acute contact dermatitis, (2) chronic dermatitis, (3) neoplasms, (4) pigmentation disturbances, (5) granulomas, and (6) ulcerative lesions.

Chemical compounds in dentistry associated with a dermatosis include the following:
1. Local anesthetics
2. Antibiotics
3. Disinfectants
4. Eugenol
5. Resins
6. Soaps

7. Waxes

8. Peroxides

Disinfectants should include alkaline glutaraldehydes, sodium hypochlorite, iodine compounds, quarternary ammonium compounds, and phenols. The resins include methyl methacrylate and composite resins.

The following precautions are suggested in the use of chemical compounds:

1. Do *not* allow materials to come in contact with the skin.

2. Wash the skin areas that do contact the chemical.

3. Wear gloves when possible to avoid contact with the chemical.

4. Inform all dental personnel of this problem.

Acids

A number of acids are used in dentistry. These chemicals can cause serious injury to the skin and may cause permanent and irreversible damage to the eyes, including blindness. Vapors from these chemicals may cause irritation to the respiratory system or even death. Acids used in dentistry include hydrochloric acid, phosphoric acid, sulfuric acid, and hydrofluoric acid.

Pickling solutions are usually composed of water and sulfuric acid, hydrochloric acid, or nitric acid. These solutions can be extremely hazardous and should be used with care. Acid etch solutions usually contain phosphoric acid and present the same hazards as other chemicals.

The following precautions in the use of acids are suggested:

1. Inform all dental personnel of the hazards of acids and pickling solutions.

2. Wear safety glasses and rubber gloves during their use.

3. Do not boil acids or pickling solutions, because this creates vapors and splatter.

4. Avoid dropping objects in acid solutions (this creates splatter).

5. Add acid to water when mixing (rather than adding water to acid).

6. Have neutralizing agents available in the event of a spill. Bicarbonate of soda will perform this function.

7. If acid comes in contact with skin, rinse the area with tap water for 5 to 10 minutes.

8. If acid comes in contact with eyes, rinse with tap water for 5 to 10 minutes, then obtain specialized treatment from an ophthalmologist.

9. Label all containers with any form of acid.

10. Ventilation is very important. Use acids and especially heated pickling solutions in an area with good ventilation or under a hood.

Alkaline Solutions

Alkaline solutions can cause injury to the skin and mucous membranes. They also have the potential to cause serious eye damage. Two alkaline solutions that may be encountered in dentistry are sodium hypochlorite and ammonium hydroxide. Hazards of alkaline solutions include (1) irritation of the skin and eyes, (2) vapor inhalation, which may cause severe bronchial irritation and pulmonary edema, and (3) corrosion of mucous membranes.

Suggested precautions in the use of alkaline solutions are the same as those for acid solutions.

Organic Chemicals

Many chemicals from this group are used in dentistry and include the alcohols, aldehydes, esters, and ethers. Many solvents and thinners fall into this group, as well as ethylene oxide and monomers. Those being used for dental purposes include the following:

1. Ethyl alcohol
2. Isopropyl alcohol
3. Methyl alcohol
4. Chloroform
5. Ethyl ether
6. Acetone
7. Benzene
8. Ethylene oxide
9. Methyl methacrylate
10. Toluene
11. Carbon tetrachloride
12. Methylene chloride

NIOSH has identified some of these chemicals as occupational carcinogens. Benzene has been confirmed as a carcinogen, and chloroform and carbon tetrachloride are suspected carcinogenic agents.

Other hazards related to use of organic chemicals include the following:

1. Contact dermatitis.
2. Nausea, vomiting, and abdominal pain.
3. Irritation to the eyes and respiratory tract.
4. Headaches and drowsiness.
5. Liver and kidney damage.
6. Hallucinations, coma, and death (in high concentrations).
7. Possible mutagenic changes.

This is a very general listing of hazards for these chemicals as a group.

Hazards associated with any particular chemical can be found in *Occupational Diseases: A Guide to Their Recognition* (published by NIOSH, U.S. Government Printing Office).

Chloroform

Chloroform is used in an endodontic procedure known as the gutta-percha–chloropercha technique. Eucalyptol (eucalyptus oil) can be used in place of the chloroform in a technique called gutta-percha–eucapercha. The transition to eucalpytol may be preferable because of the legal complications that could possibly arise from the use of choloroform. The legal complications may stem from the following statements and findings on chloroform:

1. Chloroform has been identified as a suspected carcinogen by NIOSH.

2. NIOSH recommends that chloroform be regulated as an occupational carcinogen.

3. National Cancer Institute studies involving oral doses of chloroform have demonstrated liver cancer in laboratory animals.

4. Chloroform has been deleted from *Accepted Dental Therapeutics* by the ADA Council on Dental Therapeutics.

Methyl Methacrylate Monomer

This chemical compound is singled out for discussion because of its wide use in dentistry. The vapors do not-appear to produce any long-term effects such as carcinoma. There appears to be little or no cumulative action. However, extremely high concentrations may cause unconsciousness and death. This is not likely to occur, because the odor of the monomer acts as a good warning sign. Some of the effects of exposure include irritation to respiratory tract, irritation to the eyes, decreased gastric motor function, and contact dermatitis.

The following precautions in the use of organic chemical monomer are suggested:

1. Inform the dental staff of the hazards associated with the use of these chemicals.

2. Ventilation is very important. Work in a well-ventilated area. If this is not possible, use a supplied air respirator to avoid breathing the vapor. The use of a chemical vapor hood may be desirable when using large amounts of these chemicals.

3. Wear safety glasses.

4. Wear rubber or surgical gloves.

5. Clean up any spills. Be sure to provide adequate air exchange in the area of a spill.

6. Keep these chemicals in a closed container.

7. Clean chemical off the container after each use, so that the next user does not become contaminated.

8. Prohibit smoking, eating, or drinking in work areas where these chemicals are used.

9. Thoroughly wash any areas of skin contact.

Beryllium and Nickel

Beryllium and nickel are used in some partial denture alloys as well as in some crown and bridge alloys. Both of these metals pose considerable health risks, particularly to the laboratory technician whose job involves grinding and polishing these alloys. The hazards associated with these metals are illustrated by the following:

1. NIOSH has identified nickel as a confirmed occupational carcinogen and beryllium as a suspected carcinogen.

2. There is a high incidence of lung and nasal cancer among nickel workers.

3. Nickel is a powerful sensitizer, causing more cases of contact dermatitis than all other metals. Beryllium also causes contact dermatitis.

4. Beryllium and its compounds are highly toxic and may result in respiratory irritation accompanied by pain, shortness of breath, cough, and weight loss.

5. Chronic beryllium disease can lead to a severely disabling condition characterized by extreme weakness and weight loss.

The following precautions relative to use of beryllium and nickel are suggested:

1. Use an alloy that does not contain nickel or beryllium.

2. Determine if an alloy contains nickel or beryllium. If an alloy containing these two metals must be used, then the following recommendations are offered:

    a. Inform all personnel of the hazards.

    b. Ensure adequate ventilation in the work area.

    c. Use a suction system for any grinding or polishing of these alloys. Suction should be vented to the outside.

    d. Wear gloves and a face shield.

    e. Change to uncontaminated clothing before leaving work. Ensure proper handling and washing of contaminated clothes.

    f. Any skin areas that come in contact with the alloy particles should be thoroughly washed.

    g. Prohibit smoking, eating, and drinking in the work area.

    h. Use warning label and signs on containers with these alloys and on equipment where these alloys are worked.

Gypsum Products

Plaster, dental stone, and improved stone are made from gypsum. Gypsum is another term for calcium sulfate, which may also be used in investment materials along with other chemicals and materials. The dust produced from grinding any of these materials may be hazardous to the respiratory system. A suction system at the work bench where grinding occurs will effectively control the dust and alleviate this problem.

However, the calcium sulfate may present another hazard. When it is heated above 700 degrees Centigrade, it will decompose and emit sulfur dioxide (SO_2) and sulfur trioxide (SO_3).

Hazards related to SO_2 include irritation of mucous membranes of the upper respiratory tract resulting in dryness and cough and irritation of the eyes. Prolonged exposure may result in altered sense of smell as well as fatigue and nasopharyngitis. The symptoms of chronic bronchitis may also occur with exposure over a long period of time.

As a precaution, burnout ovens should be in a well-ventilated area, and there should be a hood over the burnout ovens with an exhaust vent to the outside. If this is not possible, have an exhaust fan near the ovens that is vented to the outside.

X-Ray Processing Chemicals

Solutions used for processing x-ray film may contain a number of chemicals. Some references indicate that the ingredients responsible for toxic effects are hydroquinone (a developer) and acetic acid (a fixer). Hydroquinone is described as relatively safe in low concentrations and does not present a serious hazard. However, chronic exposure to both hydroquinone and acetic acid may have detrimental effects. Sodium thiosulfate is a major component of fixer, but is apparently not a health hazard unless it is heated to the point that it gives off toxic oxides of sulfur.

Hazards of x-ray processing chemicals include contact dermatitis, irritation of the eyes with possible staining and opacification of the cornea, and irritation of the respiratory system, including bronchitis.

The following precautions in the use of x-ray processing chemicals are suggested:

1. Ensure adequate ventilation in the work area. Good air exchange should be provided with an exhaust to vent the vapors outside the building.

2. Wear rubber gloves and safety glasses when mixing solutions, removing used solution, and cleaning tanks or automated processors.

3. A rubber apron will protect clothing from these chemicals. If clothing does become contaminated, remove and wash.

4. Keep lids on tanks and automatic processors to prevent vapor contamination.

5. Clean up chemical spills immediately to prevent vaporization.

6. Prohibit smoking, eating, and drinking in the work area.

REFERENCES

Cooley R.L., Cottingham A.J. Jr., Abrams H., et al.: Ocular injuries sustained in the dental office: Methods of detection, treatment, and prevention. *J. Am. Dent. Assoc.* 97:985–988, 1978.

Cooley R.L., Barkmeier W.W.: Prevention of eye injuries in the dental office. *Quintessence International* 9:953, 1981.

Kuwabara T., Gorn R.: Retinal damage by visible light. *Arch. Ophthalmol.* 79:69, 1968.

Merck Index of Chemicals and Drugs, ed. 9. Rahway, N.J., Merck & Co., Inc., 1976.

Mills L., Andersen F.: Ultraviolet and microwave radiation in dentistry. *Gen. Dentistry* 29:481, 1981.

Occupational Diseases: A Guide to Their Recognition. National Institute for Occupational Safety and Health, 1977.

Occupational Health Guidelines for Chemical Hazards. National Institute for Occupational Safety and Health, 1981.

Chapter 7
Radiation Protection and Safety

Olga A.C. Ibsen, R.D.H., M.S.

RADIATION SAFETY has been a major concern of governmental health agencies as far back as 1928. At that time, one of the first agencies on the federal level was formed, the International Commission on Radiological Protection (ICRP). Since that time, numerous federal, state, and local agencies have addressed the subject of radiation safety.

The Consumer-Patient Radiation Health and Safety Act, signed into law in August 1981, is the most recent document of federal legislation on the issue. This document has no doubt demonstrated the fact that legislators, consumers, and professionals are genuinely concerned about radiation protection. The federal government has established minimum standards for state health agencies to use as a guide in establishing certification and accreditation to programs in various health professions that involve exposure of patients to radiation for diagnostic or therapeutic purposes (see *Federal Register* in reference list).

In the dental profession, standards have been formulated by the Department of Health and Human Services (as mentioned in the publication cited above) for the dental hygienist and dental assistant. Dental hygienists, by nature of the fact that they are already graduates from an accredited program, are considered to have met these standards. The section addressing standards for the dental assistant states that "educational programs by an organization recognized by the United States Department of Education" are also regarded as having met these standards. Ironically, patient and operator protection does not end with the education of the operator. The dentist becomes solely responsible for the optimal radiologic practices carried out in his office. Every effort should be made to reduce the amount of exposure not only to patients, but to the clinicians or operators involved. Modern equipment, fast film, lead-lined collimaters, and precision holders are a few guides to optimal radiologic health practices for the patient. However, at the same time, these factors contribute to the optimal protection of the operator.

Dental Relevance

This chapter will explore methods of operator protection and refer the reader to various sources that, if implemented, will greatly reduce the exposure of the operator to ionizing radiation in dentistry. The dentist, dental hygienist, and dental assistant are all "operators" of the dental radiographic equipment.

Excessive exposure to ionizing radiation from the primary beam has produced changes in cell structure, chemical changes in the cell, mutations, somatic and genetic effects, and malignant transformation of cells. The most sensitive cells in the body to ionizing radiation are genetic and blood-producing cells. Continuing to the least sensitive are young bone, glandular tissue, skin, muscle, and finally nerve and adult bone.

In the dental setting, the operator is exposed to scatter radiation. There are guidelines that should be followed to assure the operator optimal protection. These will be discussed under "Preventive Measures" later in the chapter.

Detection Methods

Laboratory Tests

Blood tests such as leukocyte counts can be used to demonstrate overexposure to ionizing radiation. However, the amount must exceed 50 R to the hemopoietic tissue, and this is highly unlikely in dental settings. Even if an operator should be exposed to this amount of radiation, leukocyte counts must be performed *regularly*. If this is not done, the decrease in white blood cells could go unrecognized, because after a short period of time the number of leukocytes can return to normal levels.

Air Samples

Periodic air samples can be taken only when radioactive materials are in use. Therefore, this method of detection is not applicable to ionizing radiation in dentistry.

Area Monitoring

The Young X-Ray Radiation Detector (available from Young Dental, Maryland Heights, Mo.) is capable of measuring background and scatter radiation up to 450 mR. This piece of equipment can be used in the dental office.

Observation of Personnel in the Dental Environment

Although the operators should practice preventive techniques and safety measures, it is also important that the secretary, office manager, receptionist, laboratory technician, and any other dental staff be monitored. Work positions of these individuals should never be situated in an area where they may be in the primary beam of the radiographic equipment. Occupational exposure for radiation workers (for total body) is 5 R per year. According to the National Council on Radiation Protection and Measurements, "During the entire gestation period, the maximum permissible dose equivalent to the fetus from occupational exposure of the expectant mother should not exceed 0.5rem." Pregnant operators should be advised of this.

Symptoms and Clinical Features of Radiation Toxicity

One of the early clinically visible signs of excessive exposure to ionizing radiation is the skin erythema effect, or clinical symptomatic reddening of the skin. For the erythema effect to take place, 100 R to a specific area at one time from the primary beam must be administered. Considering that a patient receives 2 to 3 R from a full mouth series of dental x-rays, it is highly unlikely that an operator functioning along the recommended preventive guidelines could ever be in danger of receiving this kind of dosage.

Advanced signs of radiation toxicity documented in the past include ulceration of the operators fingers when the operator daily held the film in the patient's mouths over a period of many years; changes in blood-producing organs and cell structure, and linkage of dental radiography to malignancy. However, there is nothing absolutely documented in the literature that establishes a cause-and-effect relationship between exposure from dental radiographs and malignancy. Most information is hypothetical and addresses low-level radiation in general, which happens to include medical and dental radiography for diagnostic purposes.

Preventive Measures

National Council on Radiation Protection and Measurements Report 35

A booklet published and distributed by the National Council on Radiation Protection and Measurements (NCRP) explicitly outlines the guidelines for radiation protection in dental practice and includes information on installation of equipment, barriers, monitoring, and dose tables for operators. This $3 booklet is a very valuable reference source to the dentist setting up a practice. Following the recommendations and measurement guides listed, the dentist can determine the installation requirements of his equipment.

Recognized Agencies

The following agencies can provide valuable information on radiation protection:

1. Federal agencies

   - International Commission on Radiological Protection (ICRP)
   - National Council on Radiation Protection and Measurements (NCRP)
   - Federal Radiation Council (FRC)
   - Department of Health and Human Services (through FDA)
   - Bureau of Radiological Health (BRH)
   - Environmental Protection Agency (EPA)
   - Department of Transportation (DOT)
   - Department of Labor (through Occupational Safety and Health Administration—OSHA)
   - Department of Interior (through Mining Enforcement and Safety Administration—MESA)

2. State health departments
3. Local health departments (county and city)

Implementation of the material provided by these bureaus can assure the operator and patient of optimal radiologic health practices.

State and Local Health Codes

Upon installing his radiographic equipment, the dentist must comply with state or local guidelines. The key term in compliance with the guidelines is ALARA (as low as reasonably achievable). Each state has a health agency responsible for inspecting dental equipment, usually the Department or Bureau of Radiation Control. Dental x-ray surveys are conducted every 2 to 3 years, depending upon the state requirement. Dental equipment in a hospital setting is surveyed more frequently. The local health code is usually very similar to the state health code. The local code may be more restrictive, but not less restrictive. In each state, however, one factor is constant, and that is the permissible dose levels.

The following material is taken from the New York City Health Code, "Article 175: Radiation Control, Section 175.59: Dental Radiographic Installations," and should be used as a guide to optimal radiation protection.

Compliance with the code itself is not only obligatory, but truly protects the operator and the patient. It is important to note that the word "shall" in any section of this code means that the procedure is mandated.

A. *Equipment*
1. The protective tube housing shall be of diagnostic type.
2. Diaphragms or cones shall be used for restricting the useful beam to the area of clinical interest.
3. For intra-oral radiography the diameter of the useful beam, at the face of the patient, shall not exceed three inches.
4. A cone or spacer frame shall provide a source-skin distance of not less than seven inches with equipment operating above 50 KVP.
5. The exposure switch shall be of the dead-man type, and where protective barriers are required shall be so arranged that it cannot be operated outside the shielded area.
6. Each installation shall be so arranged that the operator can stand at least six feet from the patient and the x-ray tube, and well away from the useful beam during exposure. A protective barrier shall be provided where the operator cannot stand at least six feet away from the patient and the x-ray tube and well away from the useful beam during exposures.
7. The tube head shall remain stationary when placed in the exposure position.

B. *Conditions for Operation of Equipment*
1. The film shall not be held by the operator during exposure.
2. Only the patient shall be in the useful beam.
3. Neither the tube housing, pointer nor cone shall be hand-held during the exposure.
4. Only persons required for the radiographic procedure shall be in the radiographic room during the exposure.
5. For extraoral radiography, the x-ray film used as the recording medium during the x-ray examination shall show substantial evidence of cut-off (beam delineation).
6. Gonadal shielding of not less than 0.5 mm lead equivalent shall be used for patients who have not passed the reproductive age during radiographic procedures in which the gonads are in the useful beam.
7. All film used for intraoral dental radiography shall be of ANSI Speed Group "D" or faster. All developing and processing chemicals and systems shall be compatible with the film used and shall not effectively decrease the speed of the film as designated by the film manufacturer.

C. *Panoramic Installations*
   Panoramic installations are dental installations which consist of a tube head with a collimator providing a narrow (1–2-mm) useful beam and an extraoral film carrier which are interlocked in their motion about the patient.
1. Equipment
   (i) The protective tube housing shall be of diagnostic type.
   (ii) Diaphragms or cones shall be used for restricting the useful beam to the area of clinical interest and shall provide the same degree of protection as is required of the tube housing.
   (iii) A device shall be provided to terminate the exposure after a preset

time interval or exposure. The exposure switch shall be of the dead-man type.

(iv) Each installation shall be provided with a protective barrier for the operator or shall be so arranged that the operator can stand at least six feet from the patient and the x-ray tube, and well away from the useful beam.

2. Conditions for Operating Equipment
(i) Only the patient shall be in the useful beam.

Radiation Monitoring

The thermoluminescent dosimeter (TLD) or film badge is usually used to monitor dental personnel. There are advantages and disadvantages of each monitoring system that may contribute to the selection of the particular monitor.

The TLD is not as sensitive as the film badge to environmental effects such as humidity, light, or organic vapors, and it can be worn for several months at a time. It is composed of lithium fluoride crystals, which are heated to produce a particular light response when reading the monitoring device. The only disadvantage of the TLD (which really does not contribute to the decision for selecting the monitor) is the fact that a permanent record of the original reading cannot be repeated. Unlike the film in the film badge that can be reviewed repeatedly, once the TLD crystals are heated and processed for reading they are useless. In addition, the film badge must be returned monthly, because it is very sensitive to the thermal environment.

In any case, all personnel in a dental setting where radiation is used should be monitored by appropriate technology.

The following list of monitoring services was taken from a publication of the American Nuclear Society. Companies taken from this comprehensive list were those who distributed film badges (FB) or TL, which are the most appropriate monitoring devices for dental personnel.*

- Alexander Vacuum Research, Inc., Greenfield, Mass. (FB)
- Alnor Oy, Turku, Finland (TL)
- Dositec, Inc., Framingham, Mass. (FB)
- E.I. Du Pont de Nemours & Co., Inc., General Services Division, Wilmington, Del. (FB)
- Eastman Kodak Co., Rochester, N.Y. (FB)
- Eberline Instrument Corp., Santa Fe, N.M. (TL)
- FBF, Inc., Knoxville, Tenn. (FB)

---

*This list is furnished for the reader's convenience and is not an endorsement of any company mentioned. There may be other companies with similar services not documented in this publication.

- Gulf Nuclear, Inc., Webster, Tex. (FB, TL)
- The Harshaw Chemical Co., Solon, Ohio (TL)
- R.S. Laundauer, Jr. & Co., Glenwood, Ill. (FB, TL)
- Nuclear Research Corp., Warrington, Pa. (TL)
- Nuclear Sources & Services, Inc., Houston, Tex. (FB, TL)
- Panasonic Co., Secaucus, N.J. (TL)
- Radiation Service Organization, Laurel, Md. (FB, TL)
- Teledyne Isotopes, Westwood, N.J. (TL)
- United States Testing Co., Inc., Hoboken, N.J. (FB, TL) and Richland, Wash. (FB, TL)

Patient Protection

Patient protection from ionizing radiation in the dental setting affects operator protection in the following ways:

1. Collimation: Shielded open-ended cones or rectangular collimators to narrow the size of the primary beam and film-holding devices to assure accurate technique.

2. Optimal filtration: To filter out low energy and less penetrating rays that do not contribute to the quality of the image.

3. Careful evaluation and rationale for the patient's need to have x-rays taken: "Routine" procedures or directives to personnel should be absolutely eliminated.

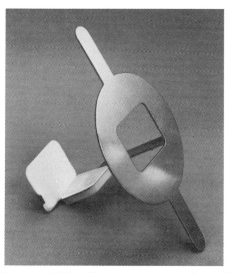

Fig 7–1.—The Precision X-Ray Device for rectangular collimation. (Courtesy of Dr. Robert Silha, Eastman Kodak Co., Rochester, N.Y., and Robert Masel, Masel Orthodontics, Inc., Philadelphia.)

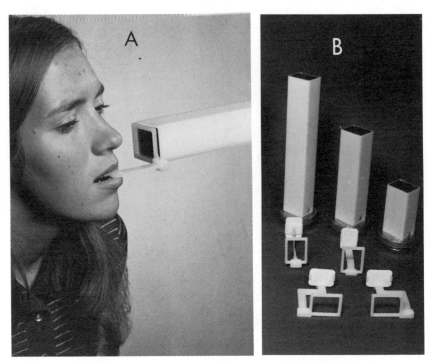

Fig 7–2.—A, B, rectangular collimators and film-positioning instruments. (Courtesy of Richard Margraf, Margraf Dental Mfg., Inc., Jenkintown, Pa.)

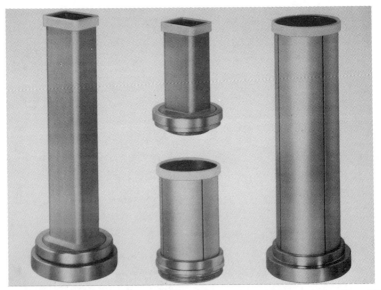

Fig 7–3.—BAI Rinn instruments for circular and rectangular collimation. (Courtesy of Nicholas Sico, Rinn Corp., Elgin, Ill.)

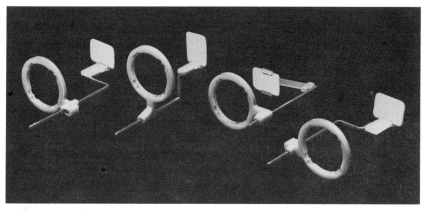

Fig 7–4.—XCP Rinn instruments for use with circular collimation. (Courtesy of Nicholas Sico, Rinn Corp., Elgin, Ill.)

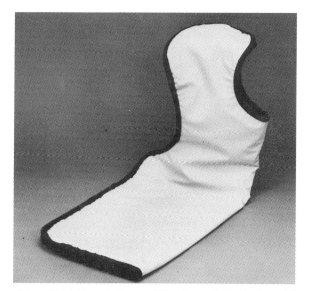

Fig 7–5.—Cling Shield Lead Apron. (Courtesy of Dr. Robert Silha, Eastman Kodak Co., Rochester, N.Y., and Gertrude Palmero, Palmero Sales Co., Inc., Stratford, Conn.)

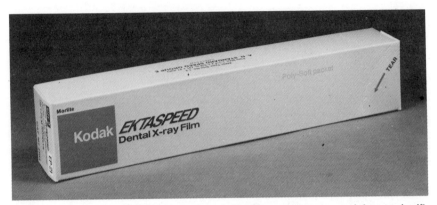

Fig. 7–6.—Kodak Ektaspeed film, for which the manutacturer claims a significant reduction in radiation exposure. (Courtesy of Dr. Robert Silha, Eastman Kodak Co., Rochester, N.Y.)

4. The highest speed film, which assures less exposure to the patient.

5. Patient shielding.

Implementation of these techniques for patient safety will expose the operator to the least possible amount of scatter radiation. This is not an assumption, but has been clearly defined in the literature. An excellent summary of how radiation is reduced and referring the reader to the sources where equipment can be purchased is provided by Robert E. Silha, D.D.S., M.S. (see reference list).*

1. The Precision X-Ray Device for rectangular collimation (Fig 7–1) (Isaac Masel Co., 3021 Darnell Rd., Philadelphia, PA 19154).

2. Rectangular collimators and film-positioning instruments (Fig 7–2) (Margraf Dental Mfg., Inc., 611 Harper Ave., Jenkintown, PA 19046).

3. BAI and XCP Rinn instruments, circular and rectangular collimation (Figs 7–3 and 7–4) (Rinn Corp., 1212 Abbott Dr., Elgin, IL 60120).

4. Fitzgerald Film Holder (Rocky Mountain Metal Products Co., 1450 Galapago St., Denver, CO 80204).

5. Cling Shield Lead Apron (Fig 7–5) (J. Palmero Sales Co., 120 Goodwin Pl., Stratford, CT. 06497).

6. Kodak Ektaspeed film, for which the manufacturer claims a significant reduction in radiation exposure (Fig 7–6) (Eastman Kodak Co., Rochester, NY 14650).

---

*Most of these references are documented in this particular manuscript, and the sources listed are not inclusive. It should be noted that the inclusion of these references is strictly for the convenience of the reader and does not carry any endorsement of these products.

7. Dental x-ray mounts, shields, etc. (Ada Products, P.O. Box 17709, Milwaukee, WI 53217).

8. Patient and operator shields (Parkell, Farmingdale, NY 11735).

SUGGESTED READINGS

The following references address radiation protection and safety.* The Bureau of Radiological Health, under the Department of Health and Human Services, provides excellent information on various aspects of radiation and how it affects the dental profession. Some of these sources are listed. There are hundreds of manuscripts published every year in various journals, magazines, and written media on the subject of radiation protection. For one of the most comprehensive treatments of this subject, see Alcox.

Administratively Required Dental Radiographs, FDA 81–8176. U.S. Department of Health and Human Services, Bureau of Radiological Health, 1981.

Alcox R.W.: Biological effects and radiation protection in the dental office. *Dent. Clin. North Am.* 22:517–532, 1978.

An Overview of Dental Radiology. U.S. Department of Health and Human Services, Bureau of Radiological Health, 1980.

Barr J.H., Stephens R.G.: *Dental Radiology: Pertinent Concepts and Their Applications in Clinical Practice*. Philadelphia, W.B. Saunders Co., 1980.

Basic Radiation Protection Criteria. National Council on Radiation Protection and Measurements, Report 39. U.S. Department of Health and Human Services, Bureau of Radiological Health, 1971. Reprinted 1974.

Comparison of Radiation Exposures from Panoramic Dental X-ray Units, FDA 77–8009. U.S. Department of Health and Human Services, Bureau of Radiological Health, 1976.

DeLyre W.F.: *Essentials of Dental Radiography for Dental Assistants and Hygienists*, ed. 2. Englewood Cliffs, N.J., Prentice-Hall, Inc., 1980.

Dental Exposure: Normalization Technique: "Dent" Instruction Manual, FDA 76–8042. U.S. Department of Health and Human Services, Bureau of Radiological Health, 1976.

Frommer H.H.: *Radiology for Dental Auxiliaries*, ed. 2. St. Louis, C.V. Mosby Co., 1978.

Goaz P.W., White S.C.: *Oral Radiology: Principles and Interpretation*. St. Louis, C.V. Mosby Co., 1982.

Manson-Hing L.R.: *The Fundamentals of Dental Radiology*. Philadelphia, Lea & Febiger, 1979.

Section 5506. *Am. Nucl. Soc. News* 25:250, 1982.

Shapiro J.: *Radiation Protection: A Guide for Scientists and Physicians*, ed. 2. Cambridge, Mass., Harvard University Press, 1981.

---

*This list of references is not all inclusive and does not constitute an endorsement of the publishers or authors.

Silha R.E.: The new Kodak Ektaspeed dental x-ray film. *Dent. Radiogr. Photogr.* 54:32–35, 1981.

Standards for the accreditation of educational programs for and the credentialing of radiologic personnel. *Federal Register* 48:31966–31975 (July 12), 1983.

Uranium in Dental Porcelain, FDA 76–8061. U.S. Department of Health and Human Services, Bureau of Radiological Health.

Wuehrmann A.H., Manson-Hing L.R.: *Dental Radiology,* ed. 5. St. Louis, C.V. Mosby Co., 1981.

Chapter 8

Conservation of Hearing for the Dentist

Maurice H. Miller, Ph.D.

NOISE IS by far the most omnipresent noxious contaminant in the work and nonwork environment. Despite its effects on virtually every American, little attention has been paid to the dangers of noise, and relatively small amounts of money have been spent to control it compared to such other threats to our environment as water or air pollution. Apart from an unnecessary and unrealistic concern with removal of wax from their external auditory canals, most persons could not care less about preservation of auditory function and are unwilling, for the most part, to take the necessary steps to protect and preserve this vital function.

To the scientist, noise is an unwanted disturbance occurring within an audible frequency band that interferes with human communication. To the acoustician, it is an erratic, intermittent, or statistically random oscillation. To the person in his workplace, excessive noise causes ringing in the ears, hearing impairment, irritability, headaches, and difficulty in communicating with others. To adolescents, the sound of rock music blaring from a stereo set may be music to their ears, but to parents and neighbors, it may be noise. To all, and by standard definition, noise is unwanted sound.

According to the National Occupational Hazard Survey, noise in the workplace accounts for 28% of the probable occupational diseases. Noise affects virtually every area where people work or play. The worker, after 8 hours of exposure to potentially hazardous noise, continues to be exposed to various avocational sources of noise that can also damage hearing. Often, he uses personal earphones attached to stereo listening sets at potentially hazardous levels on his way home from work. He may then fire hundreds of rounds of ammunition at his local hunting club. His hearing may also be affected by hundreds of factors including, but not limited to, ototoxic drugs, age, sudden deafness associated with viral and vascular factors, tumors, and heredity. He may enter adulthood with ear and auditory damage secondary to a variety of bacterial and viral diseases in childhood, including mumps, measles, and scarlet fever.

Large- and small-arms exposure, and rock, disco, and stereo music in the home and in the rock concert hall are some of the high-intensity, potentially hazardous noises to which the population is exposed. Snowmobiles, power tools, chain saws, motorcycles, and power lawn mowers also contribute to avocational noise-induced hearing loss. Noise exposure now involves over 130 million urban dwellers and 182 million automobile drivers, representing overlapping populations producing multiple sources of noise exposure. There are at least 9 million homeowners living in over 200 square miles who are exposed to subsonic and supersonic aircraft, a number that increases significantly each year.

Many potentially hazardous levels of noise are found within the home. Appliances that make life more comfortable and convenient produce high-level noises, particularly as these electronic devices age and components become worn. A blaring radio can reach a sound pressure level (SPL) of 110 dBA; an electric razor, 107 to 116 dBA; a crowd at a hockey game, 120 dBA; subway noise, 90 to 114 dBA; and a farm tractor, 120 dBA. Blenders, garbage disposal units, vacuum cleaners, and hair dryers and blowers are among the "conveniences" of modern living that expose us to brief but high noise levels.

Detection Methods

The basic instrument for measuring the physical characteristics of noise is the sound level meter, the various weighting networks of which simulate the response of the normal human ear at different frequency and intensity levels. The intensity or magnitude of the sound waves measured by the sound level meter is expressed in decibels. The decibel is a dimensionless, logarithmic unit for expressing the relative intensity of sounds on a scale from 0 to 150. Decibels are not linear units like miles or pounds. Rather, they are representative points in a sharply rising curve. Thus, while 10 dB is ten times greater in intensity than 1 dB, 20 dB is 100 times greater, 30 dB is 1,000 times greater, and so on. Sound equal to 100 dB is 10 billion times as intense as 1 dB. While 90 dB is equal to the sound of a train roaring into a subway station, 100 dB equals the sound of ten trains pulling into the station simultaneously, and 110 dB represents 100 trains.

Measures of individual hearing are made by means of a pure-tone audiometer. These tests present individual sound frequencies at SPL that can be accurately controlled. The subject indicates to the tester when the tone is just audible. The level at which the subject responds to each tone is compared with that of a normal-hearing listener on whom the audiometer has been calibrated.

The graph of audiometric testing that emerges after years of noise exposure will have strong similarities to that associated with a temporary threshold shift. The early stages of noise exposure for a group of workers is shown in Figure 8–1. The top curve shows hearing at punch-in time, while the lower curve shows the audiogram at quitting time. Note that the greatest shift appears at 4,000 Hz, with hearing approaching a normal level (but not shown) at 8,000 Hz, a characteristic of the early effects on hearing of noise exposure. Figure 8–2 shows the progressivity of hearing impairment characteristic in high noise level industrial workers who do not consistently use personal hearing protective devices.

Damage from noise exposure affects the inner ear, specifically the receptor hair cells of the organ of Corti, which is comprised of three or four outer rows of about 20,000 hair cells and an inner row of about 3,500 hair cells located on the basilar membrane in the cochlear canal. These delicate, microscopic hair cells undergo damage from what is believed to be an initially reversible biochemical saturation explaining the temporary threshold

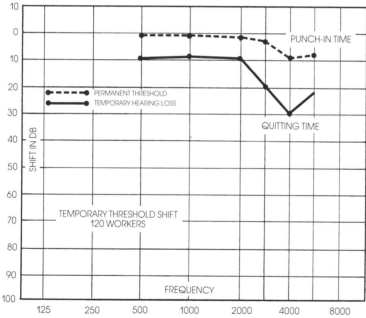

Fig 8–1.—Early stages of noise exposure for a group of workers. Upper curve shows average hearing thresholds of workers at punch-in time. Following 8 hours of workplace noise, their hearing levels have dropped to those shown in the lower curve. By the following morning, the hearing of most workers will return to the preexposure punch-in levels. The difference between these curves is the noise-induced temporary threshold shift. (From Glorig A.: *A Noise and Your Ear.* New York, Grune & Stratton, 1958, Used by permission.)

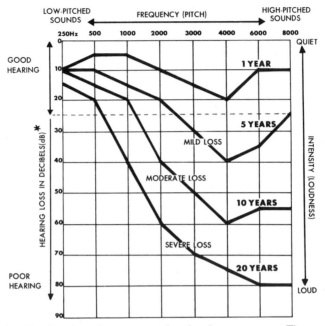

Fig 8–2.—Hearing loss from occupational noise exposure. The progressive noise-caused hearing loss in high noise level workers who do not use personal protective hearing devices results in raised hearing thresholds (the degree of loudness required for sound to be heard).

shift. Actual destruction of these sensory elements later occurs, with the outer rows of hair cells affected first. The ultimate impairment is permanent, ranging from slight disability to severe and handicapping hearing impairment. Destroyed inner ear structures cannot be surgically repaired or replaced. It is too late to decide to protect one's hearing after hair cells have been destroyed.

Noise Exposure in the Workplace

Noise may be viewed as occurring in two broad areas of life, i.e., in and out of the workplace. Since many Americans work and live in environments in which high noise levels are present, they are exposed to the cumulative and interactive affects of multiple souces of noise as well as to a vast array of nonnoise-induced contributors to hearing impairment.

Excessive noise in the workplace is of special significance as a major contributor to hearing impairment because the worker is noise-exposed for extended and continuous time periods, usually an 8-hour shift over the 40-

year average lifetime of employment. Over 5 million individual work areas in the United States are estimated to have noise levels capable of damaging the hearing of workers. Over half of the work force is exposed to daily noise levels high enough to be potentially dangerous to their hearing over a period of many years.

Extra-Auditory Effects of Noise

Noise can interfere with the intelligibility of speech and the reception of auditory signals. These effects are of importance in many aspects of our lives, because we are often called upon to detect one sound in the presence of others. Workers must hear warning signals and receive messages against noisy backgrounds; the mother must hear the crying of an infant while the radio and television are blaring; telephone communication is carried on while planes fly overhead; homework is done while stereos are tuned to high-volume settings; students are educated in classrooms adjacent to jet airports; and papers are read at conventions while interference occurs from inadequately sound-isolated adjacent areas. For speech to be intelligible, a signal/noise ratio of 10 dB is usually considered adequate. This means the desired signal, usually speech, must be 10 dB above the level of the interfering sounds, usually noise in some form. While this may be minimally adequate for speech comprehension, it may not represent a pleasant or comfortable listening environment and may, under certain conditions, lead to fatigue, irritability, vocal discomfort, and annoyance.

The psychological and non-auditory physiologic effects of noise on people are very difficult to document and sort out from a variety of other conditions that simultaneously impact human behavior and stress the organism. Noise has been implicated by one group or another as the cause of such varied conditions as insomnia, nervousness, inability to concentrate, marital discord, impotence, infertility, kidney and liver disease, cardiovascular disease, gastrointestinal disturbances, ulcers, vertigo, shrinkage of the thymus gland, swelling of the adrenal gland, and metabolic stress of the pituitary adrenal complex causing increased adrenocortical activity, vasoconstriction, increased pulse rate, and dilation of pupils. Some of this research is based on animal investigation and is of questionable applicability to humans. Much of it has been contradicted by other studies.

The sounds considered most important for the understanding of speech fall in the 300 to 3,000 Hz range. Hertz (Hz) is a unit of frequency equal to one cycle per second. Hearing impairments from most noise exposures usually occur first in the higher frequencies (3,000 to 6,000 Hz) and eventually spread to lower and higher frequencies.

Noise at a level well below the point at which discomfort, tickle, or pain occurs can produce significant hearing damage. Current federal regulations require the institution of a hearing conservation program when the level of noise to which the worker is exposed reaches or exceeds 85 dBA for an 8-hour period or its equivalent. Individual persons can sustain significant hearing damage at levels below 85 dBA, while some workers can be exposed to levels higher than 90 dB without sustaining demonstrable loss of hearing.

Auditory Effects of Noise

The effects of noise on the auditory system are well recognized and documented by many studies conducted throughout the world. Noise typically produces an initial temporary threshold shift (a reduction in hearing sensitivity) that recovers to normal levels when the individual is no longer exposed to the troubling noise. The temporary threshold shift primarily affects the high-frequency range of hearing from 3,000 to 6,000 Hz in the early stages. At this point, individuals tend to report tinnitus or ringing in the ears, inability to hear a watch tick on the affected sides, and difficulty understanding consonant-loaded words in a "cocktail party" listening condition.

As the noise exposure continues, the hearing loss spreads to surrounding frequencies. When 2,000 Hz is affected, the individual notes difficulty in distinguishing words that differ only in the high-frequency consonant sounds. Word groups like pin, tin, fin, and kin and tan, fan, and can are difficult to distinguish, particularly against a background of noise. This reduced sensitivity for the high frequencies is accompanied by other forms of auditory dysfunction, such as reduced intelligibility of conversational speech in a background of noise, hypersensitivity to sound above the impaired threshold, recruitment, and a reduced range of comfortable loudness. The temporary threshold shift that accompanies the early stages of chronic noise exposure prognosticates potential permanent hearing impairment.

Special Hazards to the Hearing of Dentists

There has been increasing interest and attention to the relationship between exposure to noise from the high-speed handpiece and noise-induced hearing loss among dentists. A significant variable to be considered in these studies is the vintage and condition of the handpieces. Early models produced noise primarily in the range of 8,000 Hz, while those with improved design in ball-bearing models and air-bearing handpieces with improved exhaust systems produce the greatest amount of acoustic energy in the

2,000 to 6,000-Hz range. Most of the studies that have been conducted were carried out under ideal analysis conditions with new equipment operating at optimum rotation speeds. Handpiece wear, burr concentricity, misuse, poor maintenance, and individual operatory design significantly influence the acoustic characteristics of the individual handpieces.

A number of early studies reported permanent hearing loss in dentists using high-speed dental handpieces. Taylor and colleagues reported in their study that at the position of the dentist's ear, levels slightly above 85 dB SPL for the octave band centered at 4,000 and 8,000 Hz were measured for a ball-bearing type of handpiece. They found a 5- and 7-dB drop in hearing thresholds at 4,000 and 6,000 Hz respectively. This is probably the best of the cross-sectional studies performed in which the hearing of dentists exposed to high handpiece noise is compared with that of a matched group of controls. Wetherton and coworkers conducted a 3-year study involving students and staff practitioners at a school of dentistry. They found no change for the students, but the staff participants exhibited some auditory change. Dental handpieces could not be implicated, because the changes in faculty were probably attributable to presbycusis. In contrast, the results of a 2-year study by Skurr and Bulteau that involved dental students indicated evidence of hearing damage of unknown cause in a portion of the 21- to 23-year-old participants. The students who had hearing impairment at the start of the study suffered further hearing deterioration. The authors concluded that it was difficult to assess how much hearing loss was due to turbine noise, but suggested that high-speed handpiece noise may not be innocuous to some ears. Hearing deteriorated in five students of a group of 17 who initially were considered to have normal hearing.

A longitudinal study was conducted by Hopp, who showed that there were no changes in the hearing thresholds of 61 dental students during the course of 23 weeks of training on the use of high-speed handpieces. This is one of the few studies in the literature in which the hearing of the same group of listeners was followed so that baseline audiometric thresholds were available prior to noise exposure. Ward and Holmberg tested the hearing of Minnesota dentists attending an Annual Minnesota State Dental Association Convention. Fourteen of the 156 dentists could identify a particular incident, usually involving gunfire, that they were sure had damaged their hearing. The authors concluded that there was no evidence that the high-speed drills produced more than a 5- or 10-dB loss at 6,000 Hz. These findings are similar to those of Taylor and associates, who found slight losses at 4,000 and 6,000 Hz. Ward and Holmberg conclude that while the danger to hearing from high-speed drills is small, it is not completely negligible. They note that 16 of 108 dentists under age 60 have losses that are handicapping and compensable under most statutes governing compensation for hearing loss. Most of these losses are attributable to gunfire and other sources of hearing damage in everyday life.

Most studies use high-speed dental drills functioning under optimum conditions. These findings cannot be extrapolated to malfunctioning equipment. If the handpiece becomes unusually noisy, the dentist may be exposed to a serious auditory hazard. Smith and Coles reported that a defective drill resulted in a level of 90 dB SPL in the 8,000-Hz frequency band. This drill noise caused not only annoyance, but a long-lasting tinnitus in both of the dentists who used it and headaches in one of them.

The Council on Dental Materials and Devices recommended that preventive measures for reduction of noise attenuation should be directed in three areas: (1) optimal maintenance of rotary equipment, (2) reduction of noise level in the operatory through soundproofing, acoustic ceilings, baffle drapes, resilient floors, and rational location of the compressor and other noise-making equipment, and (3) personal protection through the use of earplugs. They further recommended that practitioners concerned about potential hearing impairment from high-speed dental drills should have an audiologic examination. Noise levels in individual offices should be studied with monitoring periods of more than a week. An audiologic evaluation should be made after a typical workday and again at the beginning of the next day to observe temporary threshold shifts and apparent recovery. They further suggested annual retests of hearing sensitivity. Forman-Franco and colleagues studied the hearing of 72 dentists representing different specialties randomly selected from the dental department of a large suburban medical center. The specialties of periodontics, endodontics, oral surgery, pedodontics, prosthodontics, and anesthesiology had hearing thresholds in close agreement with those of the general practitioners. The orthodontic population superficially appeared to have the most significant loss of hearing at the high frequencies, but when adjusting this group for age and comparing them with a control population, only one specialist exceeded normal limits. These authors were thus unable to identify a statistically significant increase in hearing thresholds in either the central or high frequencies when the dentists were compared with the normal age-adjusted population. A slight hearing loss, not statistically significant, was found at 6,000 Hz in the general practitioner group.

These studies suggest that when average hearing levels for dentists using high-speed handpieces are compared with age-matched controls in carefully conducted studies, no statistically significant differences can be demonstrated, except at 6,000 Hz. However, *individual* dentists, particularly those at high risk, may show significant hearing impairments from high-speed drill exposure. Certainly, a dentist taking an ototoxic drug such as furosemide (Lasix) or large quantities of aspirin or one of the known ototoxic antibiotics is at risk for further hearing loss from the high-speed drill. Any female dentist taking an oral contraceptive should also be considered at risk. Dentists with known hearing loss of the sensorineural type from any cause should approach the use of the high-speed drill with caution and protective measures.

Dentists using high-speed handpieces should have annual hearing tests conducted under controlled conditions. Furthermore, the use of properly selected ear plugs when using the high-speed handpiece is strongly recommended following an examination of the ear to determine that no obstructive cerumen or other foreign body is present.

Preventive and Therapeutic Measures

Hearing impairments are of two major types: conductive and sensorineural. Frequently, a combination of both types exists. Conductive losses reflect problems in the ear's mechanical system, which consists of the outer ear and the chain of middle ear bones and related structures that are responsible for conducting sound waves from the external canal and middle ear to the inner ear. Conductive losses secondary to injury or disease of the outer or middle ear are potentially correctable by medical and/or surgical treatment.

In children, the primary cause of hearing impairment is some form of otitis media. Most common is serous or secretory otitis media, an accumulation of fluid in the middle ear that impairs the normal mobility of the tympanic membrane and adds abnormal mass to the chain of ossicles responsible for conducting sound vibrations to the fluid-filled medium of the inner ear. When conservative medical management fails, an incision into the ear drum is made through which a small plastic or polyethylene tube is inserted to act as an artificial eustachian tube. Food allergies are a frequent cause of recurrent, intractable cases of serous otitis media. Sophisticated audiologic procedures such as tympanometry allow the detection of noncompliant tympanic membranes before a hearing impairment is detected on a pure-tone audiogram. Tympanometry is a technique for measuring the compliance or mobility of the ear drum while air pressure in the external auditory canal is varied. Adults with serous otitis media should have the nasopharynx carefully examined by an otorhinolaryngologist for a possible malignant lesion.

Otosclerosis is the most frequent cause of hearing impairment in young adults, producing a conductive loss ranging from mild to moderately severe, although this condition can originate in the cochlea as well and produce significant degrees of sensorineural hearing impairment. A soft, spongy bone freezes portions of the stapes into the oval window and progressively renders the middle ear mechanism nonfunctional. A variety of modern microorthopedic surgical procedures have provided useful hearing to many otosclerotics who previously depended on hearing aids. The procedure, called stapedectomy, has a success rate of well over 95% in the hands of experienced surgeons operating on properly selected cases.

Wax in the external auditory meatus, tumors of the outer and middle ear, allergies, and congenital abnormalities of the conductive system are among a variety of other conditions that also may produce conductive hearing loss.

Noise causes a sensorineural hearing impairment resulting from damage to hair cells in the cochlea. Unlike conductive hearing loss, sensorineural impairment, for the most part, cannot be reversed by medical or surgical intervention. As previously explained, the early stages of noise exposure typically result in a reversible temporary threshold shift. If the individual sustains repeated exposure, if his inner ear is vulnerable to such damage, and if he does not use personal hearing protective devices, the threshold shift may become permanent and irreversible.

A point may be reached when the extent of the impairment will compromise the individual's ability to function socially and vocationally. A hearing aid and audiologic rehabilitation, which provides systemic training in auditory and visual comprehension, may be required. Noise-induced hearing loss, unlike conductive loss, is accompanied by various disturbing forms of abnormal auditory phenomenon that reduce the wearer's ability to derive early and complete satisfaction from a hearing aid. Frequency distortion (low frequencies are usually heard much better than high frequencies, a hypersensitivity to loudness, and a significant speech discrimination problem are but a few of the abnormal ways in which the auditory systems of persons with noise-induced impairment behave.

Auditory structures deteriorate from the aging process. Over 250 persons in every 1,000 over the age of 75 have auditory problems to a degree that interferes with understanding speech, especially in the presence of noise. For the aged, difficulty in discriminating speech is greater than would be predicted by the degree of reduced-hearing sensitivity for pure-tone stimuli. Persons in the fifth decade and above frequently suffer from problems of auditory processing resulting from deterioration of neural elements within the CNS. Over half of the hearing-impaired persons in the United States are over 65 years of age and experience a variety of peripheral and central auditory effects from the deterioration of the auditory system as a result of the aging process.

Ototoxic drugs, including aspirin, a number of antibiotics, and several of the diuretic agents in widespread use, are known to produce temporary or permanent sensorineural hearing impairment. Viral and bacterial diseases; sudden deafness from viral or vascular causes; familial forms of hearing impairment often occurring in association with lesions of the eyes, kidneys, heart, endocrine, or skeletomuscular system; tumors of the auditory nerve; and Meniere's disease (characterized by the classic triad of vertigo, tinnitus, and fluctuating low-frequency hearing loss) are among the other causes. There is substantial evidence from animal research that multiple causes of damage to the sensorineural apparatus may produce synergistic rather than additive effects.

Conclusion

Prevention is the key to protecting one's auditory system from the damaging effects of noise-induced hearing loss. The federal government, through the Occupational Safety and Health Administration, now requires hearing conservation programs for all workers exposed to a level that reaches or exceeds 85 dBA for a time-weighted average of 8 hours. The required program consists of noise monitoring with sound level meters and/ or personal noise dosimeters, audiometric testing on a serial basis reviewed by competent professionals, and regularly scheduled employee education programs.

Private citizens must understand the danger from the vocational noise to which they expose their auditory systems. Armed with such information, they can act to protect themselves. Hearing protection should be used on subways, at the rifle range, on the snowmobile, and when operating power lawn equipment and high-speed dental handpieces. Tinnitus that results from medication should be reported to the physician promptly so that dosage can be altered or the medication changed. Prompt care by an otorhinolaryngologist should be sought for upper respiratory infections to prevent permanent damage to the middle ear. Americans should avoid rock music concerts and especially avoid the use of personal earphones attached to stereo listening devices. Hearing should be evaluated after major illnesses and annually after age 50. Those who have sustained a socially or vocationally handicapping hearing impairment that is not medically or surgically reversible should see a certified, licensed audiologist for evaluation and learn to use the recommended forms of amplification in a program of professionally directed audiologic rehabilitation.

REFERENCES

Cohen A.: Extra-auditory effects of noise, in Olishifski J.B., Harford E.R. (eds.): *Industrial Noise and Hearing Conservation.* Chicago, National Safety Council, 1975.

Forman-Franco D., Abramson A.L., Stein T.: High-speed drill noise and hearing: Audiometric survey of 70 dentists. *J. Am. Dent. Assoc.* 97:479, 1978.

Hopp E.S.: Acoustic trauma in high-speed dental drills. *Laryngoscope* 72:821, 1962.

Keller J.: Effects of high-speed dental drill on hearing of dentists. *Dent. Abstr.* 10:694, 1965.

Morrant G.A.: Noise of air-turbine handpieces in relation to acoustic trauma. *J. Dent. Res.* 46:130, 1967.

Occupational Safety and Health Conservation Amendment: Part III (29 CFR 19N). *Federal Register*, August 21, 1981, pp. 42638-42639.

Pilot Study From the Development of an Occupational Disease Surveillance Method, PD-267, 511/4GA. National Occupational Hazard Survey, 1977.

Report of councils and bureaus, Council on Dental Materials and Devices: Noise control of the dental operatory. *J. Am. Dent. Assoc.* 89:1384-1385, 1974.

Skurr B.A., Bulteau V.G.: Dentists' hearing: The effect of high-speed drill. *Aust. Dent. J.* 15:259, 1970.

Smith A.F., Coles R.R.: Auditory discomfort associated with use of the air turbine dental drill. *J. R. Nav. Med. Serv.* 52:82-83, 1966.

Taylor W., Pearson J., Mair A.: The hearing threshold levels of dental practitioners exposed to air turbine drill noise. *Br. Dent. J.* 118:206, 1965.

Ward W.D., Holmberg C.J.: Effect of high-speed drill noise and gunfire on dentists' hearing. *J. Am. Dent. Assoc.* 79:1383, 1969.

Wetherton M.A., Melton R.E., Burns W.W.: The effects of dental drill noise on the hearing of dentists. *J. Tenn. Dent. Assoc.* 52:305, 1972.

Chapter 9

Ergonomics

Norman O. Harris, D.D.S., M.S.D., F.A.C.D.,
and Larry J. Crabb, D.D.S.

THE EFFICIENCY of operation of a dental operatory can be summed up with the following formula:

Efficiency of dental operation

$$= \frac{\text{quality} \times \text{quantity} \times \text{safety} \times \text{comfort}}{\text{time} \times \text{cost} \times \text{mental \& physical fatigue}}$$

Every action taken in the office somehow affects the quotient of this formula; in turn, any change in the quotient will affect the dentist, the dental team, and the patient. The various factors making up the formula are brought to life by the actions and interactions of the humans, machines, devices, and equipment of the dental environment. *It is the comprehensive study of these actions and interactions between man, machines, and his environment that constitutes the basis for the science of ergonomics.* For dentistry, ergonomics originally embodied a study of equipment design and machine efficiency—areas that were considered the exclusive responsibility of the dental manufacturer. Later, the study of ergonomics was extended to include time-motion studies to provide the basis for achieving a greater economy of motion and an increased work output in the dental office. Finally, such factors as safety and comfort, as well as personal and environmental health, were included, because these were equally important in human performance. Thus, ergonomics provides the basis for a sociotechnical working system that involves many disciplines, as well as providing the driving force for more efficient office operation.

Work-Oriented Problems

The first portion of this chapter will discuss the more global aspects of the various interdependent factors affecting efficient office operation, whereas the latter part will specifically focus on the more traditional application of ergonomics in the dental operatory.

133

The Machines

In a broad sense, the machines include all the instruments and equipment needed to more efficiently and comfortably accomplish tasks that would otherwise be impossible or would result in prolonged operations. For instance, in the course of a few centuries, the cutting of tooth structure has evolved from the use of finger-twirled cutting instruments to the foot engine, thence to the electric and air-driven turbines. This progress in machine efficiency has not been without problems. The present high-speed turbines, turning at 200,000 to 400,000 rpm, can eject tooth particles or even broken parts of cutting instruments at speeds of 30 to 35 feet per second—flying missiles that can penetrate the soft tissues of the patient's mouth or possibly the eyes of the dentist or assistant working close to the field of operation. Another major hazard of the air turbine is the aerosol cloud of bacteria, toothdust, and/or amalgam that is generated by the rapidly turning instrument. This aerosol cloud can rapidly spread throughout the operatory and entire dental building, exposing all personnel to either infectious pathogens or to particles so small that they are inhaled deep into the lung alveoli, where they cannot be removed by ciliary action.

These problems experienced with the turbine highlight a general rule in applying ergonomic principles, namely that for each ergonomic advance, there is usually a need to modify routine operating procedures, reconsider safety policies, alter design characteristics, or even add new armamentarium to make daily operations more effective and safe. To deal with the problems generated by the advanced air turbines, a high-volume, low-vacuum aspirator that could rapidly remove the continual flow of water coolant and concurrently reduce the hazardous potential of the aerosol cloud was developed. Finally, the dentist and the assistant were forced to wear safety glasses and masks to protect the eyes, face, and respiratory tract.

Within the broad scope of ergonomics, even the interaction of machines with other machines must be considered, because at times they, too, are incompatible. Some ultrasonic units used for prophylaxis or surgical techniques can adversely alter the programmed rhythms of heart pacemakers. This possibility dictates that the medical history form include a line for the patients to indicate whether they have or do not have a pacemaker.

Machines and devices do not have to be exotic to require a continual study of the safety factor. Even the simple hand instruments can be hazardous. A report in the literature relates an explorer becoming entangled in a gauze pad as it was being withdrawn from the bracket table, causing it to fall and impale the patient's eye. This possibility of causing major patient damage can be avoided by establishing safe and efficient handling techniques for instruments (an action that is part of ergonomics) and by providing the patients with safety glasses that can be worn throughout the dental appointment (Fig 9–1).

The explorer can also be a potential hazard to the patient when used in its usual role in caries examinations. Studies indicate that the bacteria picked up by the explorer in probing one carious area may result in the seeding of other noncarious areas with pathogenic inocula. This possibility mandates a consideration of the adequacy of sterilization of instruments used in different parts of the mouth, even under the most routine of conditions.

The Environment

The dental office is a closed area that contains (along with humans) teratogens, mutagenic agents, carcinogens, infectious agents, noxious-smelling

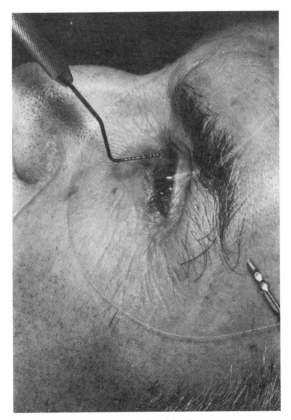

Fig 9–1.—Eye shield. A few pennies for this device may prevent eye loss and malpractice suits.

gases, possibly damaging noises, and probable lighting inadequacies. Most of these chemical and physical hazards have relatively common and innocuous-sounding names such as freon, chloroform, mercury, and asbestos. All these agents are used at times in the office or laboratory, often without knowledge that the compounds can be damaging to the health of the dental team and at times to the patients. Thus, environmental safety programs are paramount in ergonomic studies in order to capitalize on the advantages of technology, while at the same time obviating its damage potential.

Machines are also used to help solve the problems of environmental hazards. Humidifiers and dehumidifiers, heating and air conditioning are utilized to improve dental team performance and for patient comfort. Laminar air-flow air conditioning is desirable in the operatory to continually purge the environment of noxious fumes, ventilating fans are needed at appropriate locations above the laboratory benches, and amalgamators should be used in enclosed units that exhaust the mercury vapor through carbon filters.

The Humans

The machines and environment must be developed in order to support human habitation and operation in the dental office. Fortunately, the machines and the environment can usually be constructed and altered to meet human demands; unfortunately, it is the human who is the most unpredictable factor of the machine-environmental-human interface.

The social and professional actions and interactions of the members of the dental team with the patient and with each other greatly influence the amount of mental and physical fatigue generated during the daily operation of the dental office. The policies established by the dentist can directly affect these factors, and often these policies prove to be the dentist's own worst tormentor. As a common example, in the simultaneous effort to pay off past debts for education and opening an office, meeting monthly expenses, fulfilling expectations of a personal lifestyle, as well as providing for future family security, the dentist will often accept a continuing and excessive daily patient workload. This is exemplified by the findings in a study of 141 dentists by Hill and associates, in which the average number of patients seen ranged from 0.93 to a high of 3.5 per hour. In the constant effort to keep up with the accelerated time schedule, the high workloads can lead to chronic fatigue and continual stress. Over a period of time, a lower quality of work ensues, which in turn effects the efficiency of operation quotient. Also, as appointment times are shortened to compensate for patient overload, a point is reached where the patients' benefits are not commensurate with their total round-trip time commitment in coming to and going from the dental facility. The time and cost in the efficiency of operation formula are as critical to the patient as they are to the dentist.

Solutions

There are solutions to many of these work-oriented problems, which can range from the obvious action of reducing the patient load (which can often result in substituting financial stress for work stress) to a more astute employment and training of the dental team to insure better competency and compatability with the dental team members and the patients. Other readily apparent solutions include such actions as shortening office hours, taking time off for meals during the day, not taking office problems home, and engaging in off-hours recreation that is mentally relaxing.

Many of the actions that cause mental fatigue are also conducive to physical fatigue. Long working hours, an overload of patients, and inefficient patient flow all cause physical fatigue. However, even in the best-organized offices where efficient work routines are practiced, physical and mental fatigue may be generated. Attention can now be directed to these *routine* sources of fatigue as the machines, humans, and environment come together in the operatory.

Working Position of the Dentist

Until the early 1970s, the dental chair was designed for the patient to be treated in an upright sitting position; in turn, the dentist treated the patient from a standing position. A considerable expenditure of muscular energy was required to simply maintain balance in a standing position. Often the dentist of the stand-up era worked without auxiliaries or did not delegate duties if assistance was present. These practices greatly increased fatigue. An estimated 60% of a dentist's time is wasted if auxiliaries are not used. In the standing position, there was often a need to lean awkwardly over the chair. The normal standing posture was often further compromised by the need for one foot to continually search for the rheostat lever on the floor, thus putting most of the body weight on the remaining foot. One study by Buth and Klinke estimated that the standing dentist assumed a forced attitude for approximately 38% of the time. Over the years, these contorted positions resulted in circulatory and musculoskeletal problems. Varying degrees of scoliosis, kyphosis, or lordosis were common among the older and retired practitioners. The standing position also resulted in varicosities as well as leg and foot problems. The slow speed and greater torque of the belt-driven engine required a much firmer finger rest, which in turn resulted in arm and finger fatigue, plus an increase in mental stress during cutting operations. This was a hard life. In a series of studies by the ADA Bureau of Economic Research and Statistics in the early 1960s, approximately one half of the dentists retiring after age 65 did so because of ill health.

Sit-Down Dentistry

In an effort to reduce the physical fatigue of standing, dental stools began to appear in increasingly greater numbers in the 1950s. The early stools were single pedestal units, where the two legs of the dentist served to complete a tripod. They were designed for treating the upright sitting patient. Balancing on this relatively high stool, which rotated and tilted, often proved dangerous, with the stool at times slipping out from under the dentist.

It was not until the late 1960s, with development and widescale availability of the thin-backed chair in which the patient could be treated in a supine position, that a comfortable and safe stool for accomplishing four-handed dentistry was introduced to the dental profession. Sitting provided a more stable position for precision work; it also greatly reduced the muscular activity needed to maintain an erect standing position, reduced energy consumption, and created less demand on the cardiovascular system (Fig 9–2).

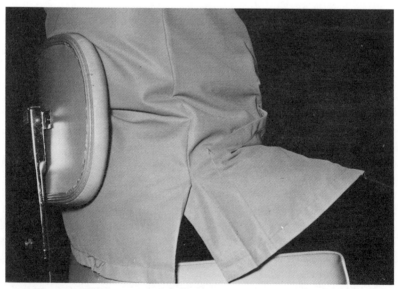

Fig 9–2.—Dentistry: a "sit-a-tory" profession.

However, the stool should not be considered the panacea to all the dentist's ailments. Many years elapsed before the hazards of the standing dentist were recognized by the dental profession. Similarly, it will probably take many years for all the problems associated with sit-down dentistry to be identified. Some potential problems have been recognized on the basis of studies relating to the sitting position. In Magora's study of 3,316 individuals in several occupations other than dentistry, approximately 54% had lower back pain if they stood for more than 4 hours a day, 42% if they sat for more than 4 hours a day, and 3.5% if they continuously varied their sitting and standing habits. If these findings can be extrapolated to sit-down dentistry, the sitting dentist and his assistant would be prudent to at least stretch and walk around the dental office several times during the day. Even when seated, an effective stress-breaking interlude can be attained by stopping work, clasping the hands behind the back, arching the spine, and breathing deeply. This can be followed by putting the arms up in the air and flexing the fingers, which in turn is followed by some loose shoulder shrugging.

In another study of the sitting position, pressure on the vertebral discs increased as the body was inclined forward and decreased as the body assumed an erect sitting position. Disc pressure also increased as the arms were extended or lifted. Such findings would indicate that the dentist should work in a comfortable upright position with the elbows in a relaxed position approximately 2 in. below the task-area height. Also, the area for exchanging instruments with the assistant should not demand excessive arm movement, a concept which is now well accepted in four-handed dentistry, where the maximum and minimum grasp lines are approximately 16 and 12 in., respectively, from the dentist.

Guidelines for Healthy Sitting

There is no "best" sitting position for everyone. Whatever sitting habits are adopted should permit ease of body mobility and minimize the possibility of abnormal sitting positions over any extended periods of time. For example, straddle sitting, where the hips and knees are flexed at right angles to each other, puts a strain on the back. In this position, the adductors force the pelvis and the spine forward. Thus, a continual sitting posture that is abnormal can lead to the same spinal problems experienced by the standing dentist—kyphosis, scoliosis, and lordosis (Fig 9–3).

The seat of the stool should be at a height that permits the thighs to be parallel with the floor, and both feet should be flat on the floor without having to bear the weight of the body. The seat should be flat and comfortable, but not so soft as to restrict movement. It should be large enough

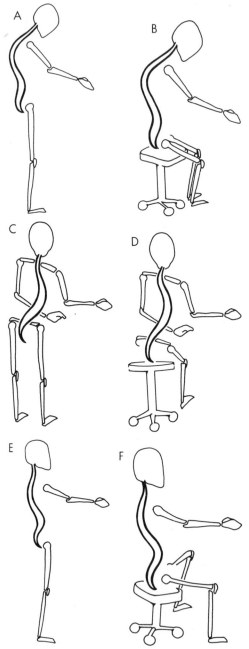

Fig 9–3.—The classic musculoskeletal problems of the standing or sitting dentist: kyphosis **(A, B)**, scoliosis **(C, D)**, and lordosis **(E, F)**.

to support the ischia, but not so deep as to cause pressure on the back of the leg. The lumbar back support should commence at approximately 8 in. above the seat, with the exact location of support varying according to the anatomy of the operator. The upper lumbar support is not as important as the lower, while too low a support does no more than push the individual forward. The wearing of loose clothing is recommended in order to avoid impairment of the peripheral circulation during long sitting periods.

In four-handed dentistry, the dental assistant must also maintain a posture that is comfortable and healthy. Because the assistant must be able to see over the operator's hands to anticipate the dentist's needs, as well as to better secure access to the mouth with the aspirator, air and water syringes, he or she must sit 8 to 10 in. higher than the dentist. In order to prevent the higher stool from tipping while the assistant is leaning forward, the stool should have a broader base with five casters instead of the four in the dentist's stool. Also, an abdominal support is needed to prevent the assistant from falling forward while performing assisting duties. The thighs can be kept parallel to the floor by supplying a ring around the base of the stool on which the feet can be supported. Like the dentist, the assistant needs lumbar support, and like the dentist, there is the potential for kyphosis, lordosis, or scoliosis if habitual contorted positions are assumed in daily routine assisting.

The sitting position is not applicable to all dental specialities. The oral surgeon and the prosthodontist, for example, must still perform most operations with the patient in an upright position. For such procedures, it is essential that the body weight be distributed equally on both feet. This can usually be accomplished, because there is now minimal need for foot activation of the floor rheostat (the major problem for the restorative dentist of the stand-up era).

Office Lighting

Paralleling the development of the thin-back chair, the modern stool, and the air turbine, office lighting also underwent a progressive evolution. From an ergonomic viewpoint, good lighting is necessary to improve the quality, quantity, safety, and comfort of dental procedures, as well as to reduce the mental and physical fatigue that are by-products of such procedures. The Castle Panovision light used from 1940 to 1960 provided one of the first commercially available shadow-free lights. Each of 28 sections acted as a reflector, directing light onto the field of vision. This light source has since been superceded by halide lights, that provide an even more intense and relatively shadow-free light. However, even these improved lights present problems. Sometimes they are not focused on the task area, a problem that is easily corrected. Of greater importance is the fact that the lights of different manufacturers have different cut-off zones below the eyes, possibly causing some patient discomfort; others differ in the intensity of light in the concentric zones extending outward from the focal point, which can cause the dentist discomfort. Even as these minor problems are being corrected by the manufacturers, there may be a need for a further reconsideration of task-area lighting. The new dental stereomicroscope, with its potential for more relaxed precision operation, does not require a unit light. Instead, two self-contained fiberoptic bundles are focused to converge on the exact work site, producing a shadow-free illumination (Fig 9–4). Following use of the stereomicroscope device, the eye adapts to light as it does when looking into a well-lighted laboratory after terminating a slide examination with a binocular light microscope.

Unfortunately for many dental offices, the planning for lighting ceases with the selection of the operating light. Yet, the task-area lighting for the oral cavity is but one aspect of the interrelated light system that is needed in an office. The task-area light source should provide approximately 1,000 to 2,000 candle power. This lighting should have a minimum color temper-

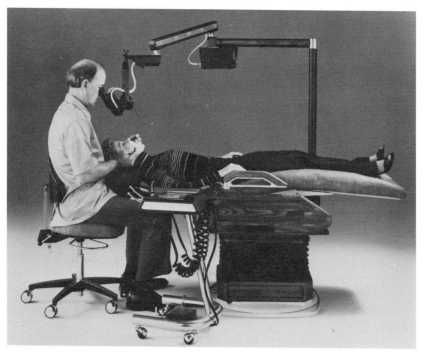

Fig 9–4.—Microdentistry permits a healthy, relaxed sitting position, with the visual field approximately 17 inches from the eyes.

ature of 5,500 degrees Kelvin for critical shade matching. Fluorescent lighting in the dental office should also have a full daylight energy spectrum. There should be a proportional relationship of the intensity (foot candles) in the task area to the area around the head and neck and to the ambient lighting in the remainder of the operatory. For instance, the illumination in the head and neck area should be from one third to one tenth the candle power of the task-area light, while the remainder of the operatory can be approximately 70 candles. This lighting relationship minimizes the amount of pupillary adaptation required for the different light intensities and thus reduces ciliary muscle fatigue. The ambient room lighting requirement prevents an excessive contrast between the dark background of the floor beneath the supine patient and the head and neck lighting.

At times, fiberoptic bundles that exit at the tip of the handpiece are used as supplementary intraoral sources of illumination. When used, precautions should be taken to maintain an adequate light level, but one that does not produce a glare that makes it difficult to adapt to a lower level of illumination outside the mouth. Another potential source of disability glare is the intense visible blue light used to polymerize some composite restorations and fissure sealants. The high-intensity light permits a greater penetration into the resin, but the illumination often causes residual visual images. Some manufacturers now provide disposable cowls that fit over the tips and are darkened around the circumference to reduce glare. The continual observation of the task area during polymerization for more than a second is contraindicated.

The patient also has to be considered in the lighting plan. Since he/she is in a supine position, the ceiling lights should be covered with a light-diffusing material that minimizes glare. Attaining this objective can also be aided by the use of tinted plastic glasses placed over the patient's eyes for safety purposes.

The above short overview of lighting relates entirely to the physical properties of light; it does not consider the possible physiologic effect of light due to the quality, rather than the quantity of illumination. In a review of light, color, and environment, Birren points out that if man were to build a community underground or under the sea, light would have to be very carefully synthesized—not merely for visual purposes, but because the quality of the light source could have an effect on life itself. Yet, many dentists practice for 30 or more years in offices that are artificially lighted at frequencies that could have adverse biologic effects. It has been reported, for instance, that red is disturbing to anxious individuals, while blue has a soothing effect. Another journal article (Paravecchio) reports the photosensitization of a patient with discoid lupus erythematosus, a result of exposure to the ultraviolet spectrum of the operatory light.

Equipment Design and Placement

The delivery of dental care demands a maximum convenient access and visibility of the task area—the mouth. This places an emphasis on the spatial relationship of the mouth of the supine patient to the hands of the dentist. Of equal importance to dentists in all specialties of dentistry is the task-area light, which permits ease of visibility. From that point, the location of all equipment and personnel in the operatory is based on the needs of the individual practitioner. For example, an operative dentist requires the immediate availability of instruments and equipment not needed by the oral surgeon, while a hygienist requires a different armamentarium than does the oral surgeon. Many of these differing specialty needs should be considered in the initial architectural design of the operatory. As the level of specialization of a dentist increases, it becomes easier for the dental architect to accurately project the needs for fixed and mobile cabinets.

There is no equipment in the dental office that is not subject to change if better function can be attained or if publicity by the dental manufacturer makes it desirable to the dental profession. The evolution of the dental chair, the operator's stool, and the air turbine have already been mentioned. The dental unit is the last remaining traditional item of the dental operatory. It, too, has undergone major changes in configuration and function. Only a few decades ago, an imposing floor-mounted unit dominated every dental operatory. It supported the dental light, a belt-driven cutting instrument, bracket table, pulp tester, air and water syringes, saliva ejector, cuspidor, and a gas burner. In contrast, the contemporary unit is a streamlined, box-like receptacle that is mainly used for housing the high- and low-torque air turbines and a combined air and water syringe. Bracket tables are now separate, while a high-volume aspirator now augments the saliva ejector. All these accessories are chair mounted.

Safety in the Dental Office

When viewed in retrospect, most accidents could have been prevented by proper foresight and planning; in reality, accidents will continue to happen, because individuals do not have the proper safety philosophy and planning to forestall their occurrence. To enlarge foresight and maximize planning to prevent the most commonly encountered accidents, every dental office should have a comprehensive safety program that is specific for *that* facility. The safety philosophy and policy should be initiated as early as possible on the basis of information derived from literature reviews, peer discussions, and individual office requirements. This safety policy should be initiated at three levels. The first level should include actions that preclude the possibility of accidents; examples of such actions would be the development of an effective standard operating procedure for sterilization or the periodic inspection of the premises for actual or developing hazards. The second level of safety planning should be directed to the immediate-response actions necessary in the event that an emergency does occur; for instance, all appropriate personnel should be trained to cope with unexpected events in responses that could range from administration of cardiopulmonary resuscitation to the expeditious use of prepositioned extinguishers in the event of fire. The third level of safety should be in the form of malpractice and comprehensive insurance in the event that a significant accident does occur involving the patient, office staff, or facility. Specific examples of the many office hazards that mandate these three levels of safety assurance will be addressed in further detail in other parts of this book.

The safety policy and standard operating procedures should be well defined in the office administrative manual. The manual should be continually updated, with all additions and problems carefully reviewed at office meetings. The review and understanding of the manual should be a mandatory requirement for the employment of all new personnel. There is a need for continual monitoring to detect program weaknesses. Reinforcement of emergency procedures necessary to cope with accidents should be accomplished on a routine schedule. All office personnel—administrators, laboratory technicians, dental assistants, hygienists, and the dentist—should be encouraged to continually *think safety* and to contribute to its office application. This safety-consciousness can often be enhanced by delegating the monitoring responsibility to office auxiliaries under the supervision of the dentist.

The existence of a comprehensive safety philosophy and policy coupled with strong support from the dentist assures a higher quality of dental care through attention to details and a greater continuing safe environment for all office personnel and patients. A much lower degree of mental stress will prevail in the office because of the realization that everything possible has been done to prevent the occurrence of an accident or at least to minimize the human or facility damage and liability in the event that an accident does occur.

Comfort

Office routines, pleasant surroundings, and compassionate people effectively performing their specialized techniques all contribute to the physical and mental comfort of the office for patients and staff alike. A few examples will be cited. For the patient, easy access to a waiting room is appreciated by the handicapped or medically compromised patient. Waiting rooms should have good lighting, and current magazines should be supplied for reading. The chairs should be comfortable to sit in, as well as easy to arise from. In the operatory, anesthetics should be used to reduce pain, while efficient four-handed techniques should be perfected to reduce both operating time and patient stress.

For the dental team, pleasant and comfortable working conditions also reduce physical and mental stress as well as increasing work output. Adequate space and efficient arrangement of equipment are needed for participation in assisting duties. Good qualitative and quantitative lighting is needed in the reception and business area, in the dental operatories and preventatories, and in the laboratory. Pleasant color schemes and background music can also help reduce the level of stress for both the patient and the dental office personnel.

Most of the examples cited are a part of good practice administration. Their inclusion in this chapter on ergonomics is to emphasize that efficiency of operation in a dental office is not solely dependent on such factors as the numbers of rpm in a handpiece, but that it is equally related to human factors within the control of the dental team. The practice of these niceties in an office increases patient tranquility and thus reduces the amount of stress transmitted to the dental team. Comfortable and pleasant surroundings enable the dental team to better cope with the physical and mental stress of the work routine, as well as to better respond to adverse patient encounters.

Relationship of Ergonomics, Physical Fitness, and Cardiovascular Problems

It has been said that the D.D.S. awarded to dental students upon graduation entitles the embryo dentist to a life of Dormancy, Degeneration, and Stress (see Cooper and Christen). The practice of dentistry is a sedentary life. Physical exertion for the sit-down dentist is mainly restricted to muscle movement of the eyes, fingers, hands, wrists, and arms. There is a demand for long hours of daily sit-down operation in one location and in one position. During that time, there is a continual need for intense concentration and precise work, both of which can be mentally and physically fatiguing. As a result of this relative physical inactivity and minimal caloric output, the dentist is often characterized as an individual with a bulging abdomen, hunched shoulders, flabby waistline, and varicose veins. This physical inadequacy has been demonstrated in one study (see Cureton) where a selected group of dentists did not perform well in physical tests, usually being below average in performance in most and above average in none. More foreboding is the fact that as the study of ergonomics continues to improve the efficiency of the office routine, there will be even less physical activity. Such a lack of body motion will result in an even greater decreased stimulus to the cardiovascular, respiratory, and musculoskeletal system.

There is a need for the dentist to compensate outside of office hours for the lack of daily physical activity experienced in sit-down dentistry. Such supplemental physical activity will permit the dentist to maintain a desirable weight, muscular tone, psychological outlook, job performance, and a cardiovascular system that will meet emergency demands. According to a study by Campbell, dentists are aware of this need for physical fitness; however, very few participate on a regular basis in physical training activities that will upgrade health status. The main reasons given in this study for lack of participation were either fatigue at the end of a workday or a lack of will. Data indicated that 27% of the participating dentists had no form of physical activity, and 72% had only 1 or more hours per week. Of this 72%, only 23% were involved in aerobic-type exercises that challenged the cardiovascular system.

In addition to demonstrating an apathy towards bettering health status, the off-hours lifestyle of many dentists appears to be directed to the acceleration of body deterioration. Smoking increases the mortality risk of cardiovascular disease and lung cancer, while high blood pressure from stress increases the probability of stroke. These, together with alcoholism and its related effects, are the most important causes for the premature deaths of dentists, which are (in order of frequency) cardiovascular disease, lung cancer, automobile accidents, cirrhosis, and stroke.

A correlation between cardiovascular disease and lack of physical activity has been demonstrated in epidemiologic studies by Fox and his coworkers. Conversely, where there is vigorous exercise in leisure time, there is a lower risk of coronary disease. Low levels of physical fitness can be increased by physical training. Studies by Boyer and Kasch indicate that physical training can lead to a reduction in blood pressure. It is essential that the escalation from poor physical condition to one of fitness be slow and progressive; the infrequent participation in vigorous physical activity is contraindicated, much for the same reason that untrained individuals involved in occasional heavy occupational work are confronted with an increased mortality risk. However, the critical need to strive for physical fitness is reflected in a 5- to 7-year follow-up study by Gyntelberg and associates relating to physical fitness and risk of myocardial infarction, in which they noted that "The data on leisure-time physical activity among 5,249 Copenhagen males, aged 40–59, and risk of coronary heart disease, indicated that only physical activity inducing a physical training effect, is related to decreased risk." Because maximum aerobic output, cardiac output, and heart rate all decline with age, exercise for individuals in their 60s should be lighter than for those in their 40s.

Probably one of the best ways to attain a high level of physical fitness is aerobic exercise. In this kind of program, several exercise options are possible, such as jogging, climbing stairs, bicycle riding, or aerobic dancing. Usually these routines consist of a 5-minute initial warm-up with calisthenics and stretching of muscles and tendons. Then a period of more intensive exercise follows, which can extend from 20 minutes of vigorous exercise, to 45 to 60 minutes for brisk walking. This is then followed by a cool-down period of another 5 minutes, where the same or different exercises are continued at a much reduced rate. After the cool-down period, the heart rate should be less than 120 beats per minute. To continually maintain this level of physical fitness, a minimum of three-times-per-week participation is required.

Summary

Dental ergonomics is a study of all those human, machine, and environmental factors that maximize the quantity and quality of oral health care: optimize the safety and comfort of the patient and dental team alike, and minimize the time investment, cost, and mental and physical fatigue for both those treated and the health professionals responsible for the delivery of oral health care.

For most dental operations involving the three most common causes for which people seek dental treatment (caries, periodontal disease, and prophylaxis procedures), dental care can be delivered from a sitting position. This sitting position for both the dentist and the assistant has evolved from the standing position as a result of major equipment modifications. If used correctly, these new features add efficiency, precision, and comfort to the work of the dental team. If used incorrectly, they can add mental fatigue and physical deterioration.

The dental environment contains hazards that can be detrimental to the patient and the dental health professional. Thus, there has been a continual ergonomic study by industry, the dental profession, and by individual dentists on how to accentuate the positive factors inherent in an efficient, safe, and healthy practice and how to eliminate the negative factors.

The importance of considering the broad scope of ergonomics becomes much more personal with the introduction of a second formula relating to the efficiency of dental operation:

$$\text{Income for a dental office} = \frac{\text{quality} \times \text{quantity} \times \text{safety} \times \text{comfort} \times \text{fee schedule}}{\text{time} \times \text{cost} \times \text{mental \& physical fatigue}}$$

The implications of this formula should justify the role of ergonomics in dental practice.

REFERENCES

Anderson J.A.: The selection and use of operator's stools and contour chairs. *Dent. Clin. North Am.*, July 1965, pp. 303–318.

Anderson B.J.G., et al.: The sitting posture: An electromyographic and discometric study. *Orthop. Clin. North Am.* 6:105–120, 1975.

Barnes R.: Hazards in the dental office. *Aust. Dent. J.* 19:4–6, 1974.

Bergen S.F., McCasland J.: Dental operatory lighting and tooth color discrimination. *J. Am. Dent. Assoc.* 94:130–134, 1977.

Birren F.: *Light, Color and Environment.* New York, Van Nostrand Reinhold Co., 1969.

Boyer J.L., Kasch F.W.: Exercise therapy in hypertensive men. *J.A.M.A.* 211:1668–1673, 1970.

Bureau of Economic Research and Statistics, American Dental Association: Survey of Dentists over 60. *J. Am. Dent. Assoc.* 67:454–457, 539–548, 1963.

Bureau of Economic Research and Statistics, American Dental Association: Survey of dentists over 60. *J. Am. Dent. Assoc.* 68:119–124, 1964.

Buth K., Klinke G.: The posture of the dentist. *Stomatol. D.D.R.* 29:68–71, 1979.

Campbell M.J.A.: An activity survey of dentists. *Aust. Dent. J.* 16:22–24, 1971.

Clausen J.P.: Circulatory adjustments to dynamic exercise and effect of physical training in normal subjects and in patients with coronary artery disease. *Prog. Cardiovasc. Dis.* 18:459–495, 1976.

Cloutman G.W.: The problem of fatigue in dentistry. *Br. Dent. J.* 114:317–321, 1971.

Cooper K.H.: *The Aerobics Way.* New York, M. Evans and Co., 1977.

Cooper K.H., Christen A.G.: Dentist, heal thyself: Modification of lifestyle. *Dent. Clin. North Am.* 22:323–338, 1978.

Cureton T.K.: Health and physical fitness tests of dentists (with implications). *J. Dent. Med.* 16:211–222, 1961.

D'Hondt D.G., Pape H., Loesche W.J.: Reduction of contamination on the dental explorer. *J. Am. Dent. Assoc.* 104:329–330, 1982.

Fox S.M., Naughton J.P., Haskell W.L.: Physical activity and the prevention of coronary heart disease. *Ann. Clin. Res.* 3:404–432, 1971.

Gennari V., Galli S.: Disorders that affect the dentist's osteomuscular system (a statistical study). *Riv. Ital. Stomatol.*26:479–489, 1971.

Glenner A.: The bright side of dentistry. *J. Am. Dent. Assoc.* 88:49–59, 1971.

Goldberg R.: Dentistry under a microscope. *Dent. Practice* 6:58–62, 1982.

Green E.J., Brown M.E.: An aid to the elimination of tension and fatigue: Body mechanics applied to the practice of dentistry. *J. Am. Dent. Assoc.* 67:679–697, 1963.

Gyntelberg F., Lauridsen L., Schubell K.: Physical fitness and risk of myocardial infarction in Copenhagen males aged 40–59: A five- and seven-year follow-up study. *Scand. J. Work Environ. Health* 6:170–178, 1980.

Harris N.O., Crabb L.J.: Ergonomics: Reducing mental and physical fatigue in the operatory. *Dent. Clin. North Am.* 22:331–345, 1978.

Hartley J.L.: Eye and facial injuries resulting from dental procedures. *Dent. Clin. North Am.* 22:505–515, 1978.

Hill P.H., Schissler B., Sampson P.B., et al.: Dentists' work habits: A survey. *J. Am. Dent. Assoc.* 81:1125–1130, 1970.

Kajland A., Lindval T.: Occupational medical aspects of the dental profession. *Work Environ. Health* 11:100–107, 1974.

Kimmel K.: Working systems in a dental environment. *Quintessence International,* December 1973, pp. 69–72.

Kimmel K.: Stress situations in dental practice. *Quintessence International,* November 1975, pp. 77–82.

Magora A.: Investigation of the relationship between low back pain and occupation. *Ind. Med.* 41:5–9, 1972.

Miller R.L.: Air pollution and its control in the dental office. *Dent. Clin. North Am.* 22:453–476, 1978.

Morris J.N., Chave S.P., Adam C., et al.: Vigorous exercise in leisure-time and the incidence of coronary heart-disease. *Lancet* 1:333–339, 1973.

Nixon G.S.: Chairside ergonomics. *Int. Dent. J.* 21:270–277, 1971.

Paravecchio R.: Photosensitization of a patient with discoid lupus erythematosis by a dental operating light: Report of a case. *J. Am. Dent. Assoc.* 94:907–909, 1977.

Pollack B.F., Lewis A.L.: Visible light resin-curing generators: A comparison. *Gen. Dentistry* 29:488–493, 1981.

Preston J.D., Ward L.C., Bobrick M.: Light and lighting in the dental office. *Dent. Clin. North Am.* 22:431–451, 1978.

Price D.L., Shaw W.A.: Illumination of the dental operatory. *J. Am. Dent. Assoc.* 98:925–928, 1979.

Report: The use of photography in studying postures and procedures. *Quintessence International,* February 1976, pp. 75–82.

Riessner F.F.: The dynamic seated position. *Quintessence International,* April 1972, pp. 73–80.

Roseman R.H., Bawol R.D., Osherwitz M.: A 4-year prospective study of the relationship of different habitual vocational physical activity to risk and incidence of ischemic heart disease in volunteer male federal employees. *Ann. N.Y. Acad. Sci.* 301:627–641, 1977.

Sellers W.R., Young J.M., Powell J.M.: *The Scientific Application of Light and Color to the Dental Environment.* U.S.A.F. School of Aerospace Medicine, Review 2–78. Brooks Air Force Base, Texas, 1978.

Tarasoff G.D.: Postural and kinaesthetic considerations in modern sit-down dentistry. *J. Can. Dent. Assoc.* 35:154–158, 1969.

Tressler D.: Varicose veins: An occupational disease of dentists. *Rev. Fr. Odonto-stomatol.* 3:1279–1286, 1957.

Vinard H.: Psychophysiology in dental practice administration. *Quintessence International,* April 1977, pp. 73–78.

Viohl J.: Dental operating lights and illumination of the dental surgery. *Int. Dent. J.* 29:149–163, 1979.

Chapter 10

Stress and Distress in Dental Practice

Arden G. Christen, D.D.S., M.S.D., M.A.

DENTISTRY IS a stressful occupation. Various studies and anecdotal reports strongly suggest that certain disorders and afflictions, especially in susceptible individuals, are directly related to the chairside practice of dentistry. American dentists themselves believe that fellow dental professionals suffer disproportionately from divorce, alcoholism, coronary heart disease, drug abuse, and suicide. A great number of dentists are experiencing significant levels of overstress leading to physical and psychic illness. Perhaps these individuals are "hot reactors" to the stresses they encounter, because evidence shows that the majority of practicing dentists are coping successfully as professionals and as human beings.

Causes of premature death among middle-aged male dentists are (in order of frequency) (1) cardiovascular disease, (2) lung cancer, (3) automobile accidents, (4) cirrhosis, and (5) stroke. They are all primarily diseases or conditions of choice and compulsion with stress as a major component and basically related to lifestyle. Interestingly, none are infectious in nature. Dentists often adopt self-destructive habits that lead to these conditions.

The purpose of this chapter is threefold: to present basic concepts concerning external stressers in dentistry and how they may be personally perceived, to review Hans Selye's theories of stress and discuss how excessive stresses can lead to psychic and/or physical illness, and to identify productive, realistic stress management and coping techniques.

Basic Concepts

Definitions: Stress and Stressors

What is stress? Dr. Hans Selye, a Vienna-born endocrinologist, professor at the University of Montreal, and the world's foremost authority on stress, invented this term about 40 years ago. As a young doctor, Selye (pronounced SEL-yay) emigrated from central Europe to Canada in the 1930s.

He borrowed the English word "stress" from physics to describe the body's response to everything from viruses and cold temperatures to emotions such as fear and anger. Selye defines stress as follows:

> Stress is the body's nonspecific response to *any* demand placed on it, whether that demand is pleasant or not. Sitting in a dentist's chair is stressful, but so is enjoying a passionate kiss with a lover; after all, your pulse races, your breathing quickens, your heart beat soars. And yet, who in the world would forgo such a pleasurable pastime simply because of the stress involved? Our aim shouldn't be to completely avoid stress. Which at any rate would be impossible, but to learn how to recognize our typical response to stress and then to try to modulate our lives in accordance with it.

His numerous experiments on animals and humans have described the mechanisms in detail, explaining the body's adaptation to stress and clarifying the interaction between the mental and physical. In common usage, the word "stress" now refers to the causes of stress, or what Selye calls "stressors," as well as the body's response. Stressors are specific agents or situations that can produce a bodily stress response. In and of themselves, they are neither good nor bad and can be physical, social, or psychological in nature. Complete freedom from these stressors is death! According to Katz (*Dental Practice* 1:59, 1980), stress has three components: (1) the situation or stressor, (2) one's perception and interpretation of the situation, and (3) one's physiologic and psychological response to the situation. Each of these components is unique for each person.

"Good" Stress (Eustress)

As the rates of heart disease and mental illness have mounted in modern industrial societies, stress has acquired somewhat of a bad reputation. Therefore, it is tempting to believe that all forms of anxiety and tension are abnormal. In spite of the overwhelming negative connotation of stress, certain kinds of stress, what Selye calls "eustress," are good for people. Moderate amounts of stress can add to the adventure, competition, excitement, and challenge of living. All humans need a certain level of stress and mental stimulation in order to lead fulfilled lives. Just being alive involves a continuous response to internal and external sources of stress. Selye believes that all the rhetoric about the dangers of overwork and excessive striving by type A personalities is, in many ways, an exaggeration and can arouse unnecessary anxiety (*Psychology Today* 11:60, 1978).

Many dentists work extremely long hours in their busy practices without becoming ill beyond the norm. They simply enjoy being stretched and positively flourish in their stresses. By avoiding stress, modern men and women may be avoiding the opportunity to better their lives. Selye firmly believes that hard work is both an obligation and, if approached in the right spirit, a pleasure. He believes that this attitude toward life should be cultivated.

This desirable type of stress is viewed as positive and useful in strongly motivated and healthy individuals, but it is controlled. For example, consider the keen rivalry experienced between opponents in athletic events. Intentional stress experienced by competitive runners or handball players is sought and usually relished, but it is framed. The competitors realize that there will be stress, but they know it will end. Good stress can accomplish the following:

1. Increase our levels of energy and vitality, preventing stagnation and boredom.

2. Act as a motivator, helping us find meaning in our existence and our work.

3. Improve our capability for productive behavior, creativity, and growth by providing increased opportunities and resources.

4. Increase personal awareness of our environment.

As Selye has stated, "Stress is the spice of life. Who would enjoy a life of no runs, no hits and no errors?" Stress is not merely nervous tension or something to be avoided. It needs to be harnessed and controlled for good. What humans need is the right kind of stress for the right length of time and at the level that is best for them. The key is not to exceed one's critical limit. Given too little stress, we rust out; given too much, we burn out.

Distress

Every era has been an age of anxiety; old stresses have been replaced by new ones. The threat of the plague during the Middle Ages is now only of historical interest to the modern-day American. The possibility of nuclear war, however, is imminently threatening. Selye believes that one type of social stress that has particularly increased in modern times and is far worse than others is purposelessness. He states, "This is a loss of motivation, a spiritual malady that has assumed almost epidemic proportions among the young. And with it, naturally, comes desperate attempts to escape the dilemma by any spastic effort. I believe that a large part, if not the major part, of violence, alcoholism, and drug addiction is due to a loss of the stabilizing support of constructive goals."

Ordinarily, experiences and emotions such as anger, joy, frustration, and love, give texture and meaning to one's life. However, emotional or physical stressors, if excessively severe, prolonged, or out of control, can take a harsh toll on the body. Distress is ultimately a "subjective psychological state which results from the individual's interpretation or perception of an event or situation as somehow threatening to one's well being—physical or emotional." Distress can occur as a result of any unsatisfactorily resolved situation, condition, or incident. It often represents a cumulative stress overload. In reality, it is not the individual stressor in and of itself that causes problems, but rather the meaning an individual ascribes to this unrelieved stress.

Many dentists enjoy a high-pressure practice. Selye would call these dentists "race horses." They thrive on responsibility, a sense of control, high activity, stimulation, challenge, and involvement, and are only happy with a vigorous, fast-paced lifestyle. Other dentists could be likened to "turtles," being designed for a peaceful, quiet, and generally tranquil environment.

Typically and incorrectly, stress is viewed as an unwanted intrusion by an external event or force that impinges on our daily lives. Under this viewpoint, we are victims of unwanted outside circumstances (Fig 10–1). Humans can react positively or negatively to excessive stresses by (1) learning how to cope successfully with the distress and developing a sense of completion, exhilaration, and self-control, (2) exhibiting emotional distress and becoming involved in a vicious cycle of escapism, (3) displaying aberrant, nonproductive forms of behavior such as inefficiency, disorganization, and immobility, and (4) developing physical symptoms of illness.

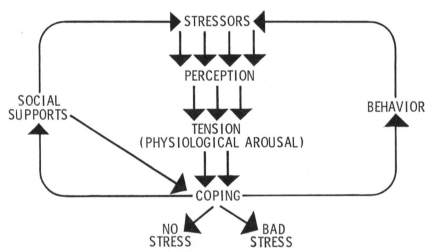

Fig 10–1.—The interrelationship between stressors, perceptions, tensions, and coping. When we use social support to let others know that we have a problem or when we exhibit appropriate behavior, it is possible to modify external stressors, thereby reducing distress. (Courtesy of Glenn Swogger, Jr., M.D., The Menninger Foundation, Topeka, Kan.)

Stressors Inherent in Dental Practice

Several studies show that chairside dentists perceive they are under a great deal of stress in their practices (Table 10–1). Interestingly, they relate few of these stresses to the technical side of dentistry. An analysis of the dental literature (Table 10–2) reveals that these external stressors are generally related to operational considerations, interpersonal relationships, or from hazards occurring in the dental office environment.

Measurement of Life Stresses

In 1967, Thomas H. Holmes and Richard N. Rahe from the University of Washington developed the Social Readjustment Rating Scale (SRRS). This 43-item list of ranked life crises or stress situations, called "life change units" (LCUs), help individuals quantitate stress levels for the previous 12 months (Table 10–3). These events pertain to major areas relating to American social structures, including the family constellation, marriage, occupation, economics, residence, group and peer relationships, education, religion, recreation, and health. The intensity and duration of change accompanying the retrospective event determined its rank value, rather than its degree of desirability or undesirability. These life events contain positive, negative, frequent, and rare occurrences.

Studies have shown that for most individuals, as the LCUs increase, so do the incidences of illness. A cluster of life changes whose values total 150 LCUs or more in a 12-month period indicate a "life crisis." At present, however, the test is not predictive of the kinds of levels of stress likely to cause illness in any given individual. Stress is idiosyncratic. It affects peo-

TABLE 10–1.—Most Common Sources of Perceived Stress as Reported by 4,033 Practicing Civilian American Dentists (in ranked order), 1978-1982

KATZ TEXAS 300 DENTISTS	GODWIN ET AL. MICHIGAN 33 DENTISTS (%)	DUNLAP ET AL. NATIONAL 3,700 DENTISTS (%)
1. Time management	1. Patient management (73)	1. Perfectionism (64)
2. Employee management	2. Business management (50)	2. Patients having pain (62)
3. Patient relationships	3. Idealism (38)	3. Sensing fear in patients (57)
	4. Staff management (33)	4. Feeling pressure to make more money (56)
	5. Time management (26)	5. Feeling others can't do things right (38)
		6. Feeling overworked or hurried (34)

TABLE 10–2.—A List of Some Potentially Destructive Stressors
in Dental Practice

Operational Stressors
- Physical immobility of dental personnel to a fixed office location and relatively restricted surrounding work area.
- Compulsive attention to cleanliness, orderliness, and perfectionistic details that are inherent in dentistry.
- The physical difficulty and mentally taxing nature of dental treatment that must be completed in a restricted, dark, wet oral area.
- The necessity of processing patients in a highly structured setting in a clockwork fashion.
- Time-pressure problems, which are inevitable even in the best-planned offices.
- Fewer opportunities for solo dentists to share experiences and relieve stresses through peer reinforcement.
- Inordinately high costs of equipping an office and coping with an overhead as high as 60% of gross income.

Interpersonal Relationship Stressors
- The constant pressure of decision making, plus the continual assuaging and counseling of complaining patients.
- Anxiety, apprehension, fear, and pain, which are frequently present in the dental situation.
- The reception of frequent overt verbal rejection from patients, e.g., "Doctor, don't take this personally, but I hate dentists!"
- The necessity to hire and fire dental office personnel.
- The necessity of the dentist to perform in a variety of societal roles for which he or she may be inadequately prepared (e.g., psychologist, salesperson, businessman, humanist, technician, personnel manager, professional, and teacher).

Office Environmental Stressors
- Physical fatigue and injuries related to the day-by-day chairside practice of dentistry, which can lead to postural defects, eye strain, varicose veins, back trouble, muscular spasms, and circulatory disorders.
- Inadequate lighting in the dental office.
- Uncontrolled or excessive sound and noise.
- Air pollution from gaseous and particulate materials, including mercury vapor and nitrous oxide.
- Eye and facial injuries generated from dental procedures.
- The spread of contagious diseases in the dental office.
- Improper control of ionizing radiation.

TABLE 10–3.—Social Readjustment Rating Scale*

LIFE EVENT	MEAN VALUE
1. Death of a spouse	100
2. Divorce	73
3. Marital separation from mate	65
4. Detention in jail or other institution	63
5. Death of a close family member	63
6. Major personal injury or illness	53
7. Marriage	50
8. Being fired at work	47
9. Marital reconciliation with mate	45
10. Retirement from work	45

TABLE 10–3.—*Continued*

11. Major change in the health or behavior of a family member	44
12. Pregnancy	40
13. Sexual difficulties	39
14. Gaining a new family member (e.g., through birth, adoption, oldster moving in, etc.)	39
15. Major business readjustment (e.g., merger, reorganization, bankruptcy, etc.)	39
16. Major change in financial state (e.g., a lot worse off or a lot better off than usual)	38
17. Death of a close friend	37
18. Changing to a different line of work	36
19. Major change in the number of arguments with spouse (e.g., either a lot more or a lot less than usual regarding childrearing, personal habits, etc.)	35
20. Taking out a mortgage or loan for a major purchase (e.g., for a home, business, etc.)	31
21. Foreclosure on a mortgage or loan	30
22. Major change in responsibilities at work (e.g., promotion, demotion, lateral transfer)	29
23. Son or daughter leaving home (e.g., marriage, attending college, etc.)	29
24. In-law troubles	29
25. Outstanding personal achievement	28
26. Wife beginning or ceasing work outside the home	26
27. Beginning or ceasing formal schooling	26
28. Major change in living conditions (e.g., building a new home, remodeling, deterioration of home or neighborhood)	25
29. Revision of personal habits (dress, manners, association, etc.)	24
30. Troubles with the boss	23
31. Major change in working hours or conditions	20
32. Change in residence	20
33. Changing to a new school	20
34. Major change in usual type and/or amount of recreation	19
35. Major change in church activities (e.g., a lot more or a lot less than usual)	19
36. Major change in social activities (e.g., clubs, dancing, movies, visiting, etc.)	18
37. Taking out a mortgage or loan for a lesser purchase (e.g., for a car, T.V., freezer, etc.)	17
38. Major change in sleeping habits (a lot more or a lot less sleep, or change in part of day when asleep)	16
39. Major change in number of family get-togethers (e.g., a lot more or a lot less than usual)	15
40. Major change in eating habits (a lot more or a lot less food intake or very different meal hours or surroundings)	15
41. Vacation	13
42. Christmas	12
43. Minor violations of the law (e.g., traffic tickets, jaywalking, disturbing the peace, etc.)	11

*The amount of life stress a person has experienced in a given period of time (i.e., 1 yr) is measured by the total number of LCUs. These units result from the addition of the values (shown in the right column) associated with events that the person has experienced during the target time period (From: Holmes T.H., Rahe R.H.: The social readjustment rating scale. *J. Psychosom. Res.* 11:213–218, 1967. Used by permission.)

ple in different ways. For example, studies show that as many as one in four of Nazi concentration camp survivors were able to resume completely normal lives in spite of the extreme distress they suffered while they were in captivity.

In January 1979, Suzanne C. Kobasa, a personality theorist and researcher from the University of Chicago, noted in her published doctoral dissertation that although the LCU concept was valid, a considerable percentage of the 670 middle- and upper-level executives she studied did not become ill even when they had high stress scores as measured by the SRRS. She identified a constellation of personality factors that characterized those persons who were more resistant to the effects of LCUs. Kobasa labeled these individuals "hardy" types. These resistant individuals possessed three general characteristics:

1. *Control:* They believed that basically, they controlled or influenced the events in their lives rather than feeling powerlessness. ("I can do it!")

2. *Commitment:* They felt deeply involved or committed to their institutions, activities, and work, rather than alienated and vegetative. ("I'm involved!")

3. *Challenge:* They anticipated change as an exciting challenge that aided their personal development and growth and were not threatened by newness or departures from old norms. ("This is a great opportunity!")

Results of Distress: The Stress Syndrome

Under any kind of stress, humans show a certain common set of physiologic defense reactions, which Selye termed the General Adaptation Syndrome (GAS).

The body reacts to all forms of stress in three stages: (1) *alarm* (defense mechanisms become activated), (2) *resistance* (stage of maximum adaptation), and (3) *exhaustion* (adaptive mechanisms collapse). For example, if a man leaps into cold water, he suffers from an initial shock, then his body begins to adapt, resisting the initial numbness. If he stays in the water too long, his body can eventually no longer bear it, and he succumbs to exhaustion.

Likewise, in the short term, humans normally are constructed to deal physically with momentary demands by fight or flight, e.g., "to throw sticks at tigers." Under these conditions, the pituitary gland releases ACTH (adrenocorticotrophic hormone) into the bloodstream, which in turn stimulates the adrenals to produce another hormone, cortisol. This causes the heart to beat rapidly and the muscles of the stomach and the intestines to contract, thus increasing the general blood circulation. Breathing speeds up as the body prepares to fight or flee.

In contemporary society, one is frequently prevented from using the fight-or-flight response because it may be socially unacceptable or prohibited. If the body is primed for action but chronically unable to act, excessive stress is not dissipated, and physiologic response systems become locked into the "on" position. This leads inevitably to a build up of frustration and pent-up emotions until the body insists that these emotions be expressed. This constant strain on the defense mechanism eventually leads to the depletion of bodily defenses, causing emotional and physical malfunctioning.

Prolonged chronic stress release leads to increased cortisol levels in the blood, which in turn trigger an increase in blood cholesterol. Catecholamine elevations have also been directly associated with myocardial necrosis, increased peripheral resistance, hypertension, and hyperglycemia. Linings of the coronary vessels can become occluded by cholesterol plaques, causing a heart attack. Other diseases and conditions related to stress overload are arthritis, alcoholism, gastric ulcer, colitis, drug addiction, insomnia, suicide, high blood pressure, and divorce. The list of physiologic and psychological problems linked to unresolved stress is almost limitless (Table 10–4).

Stress Management and Coping Techniques

Selye's Three Antidotes to the Stresses of Life

In a 1978 article in *Psychology Today*, Selye summarized 40 years of experience and scientific work in the field of stress reduction by concluding that there were three antidotes to the stresses of life.

The first ingredient, as I told you, is to seek your own stress level, to decide whether you're a racehorse or a turtle and to live accordingly. The second is to choose your goals and make sure they're really your own, and not imposed on you by an overhelpful mother or teacher. For example, I truly wanted to be a scientist; otherwise, I'm sure I would have succumbed to the pressures of my work. I've seen too many cases of doctors who really wanted to be musicians, or office clerks who really wanted to be plumbers or carpenters, not to realize how much stress is caused and suffering is involved in trying to live out the choices other people have made for you. And the third ingredient to this recipe is altruistic egoism—looking out for oneself by being necessary to others, and thus earning their good-will. I've always advised my children and students not to worry about saving money or about climbing the next rung on their career ladder. Much more important, they should work at making sure they're useful, by acquiring as much competence in their chosen fields as they can—their ultimate protection no matter what the future holds in store.

TABLE 10–4.—SUBJECTIVE PHYSIOLOGIC AND PSYCHOLOGICAL SIGNS AND SYMPTOMS OBSERVED IN INDIVIDUALS EXPERIENCING CHRONIC, UNCONTROLLED STRESS (DISTRESS)*

* Overconcern for meeting deadlines.
* Compromised treatment (preoccupied with quantity rather than quality).
* High resistance to going to work every day (clock watching).
* Chronic fatigue and exhaustion at work and at home.
* Burnout (physical and mental exhaustion of one's resources).
* Family/business problems and conflicts.
* Boredom, dissatisfaction with life in general, low motivation.
* Depression leading to isolation and social withdrawal with inability to confide in others.
* Feeling a sense of failure and being "trapped" (low self-esteem).
* Destructive ways of coping (alcohol and/or drug addiction).
* General irritability, anger, resentment, and cynicism.
* Decline in sense of humor.
* Pounding of the heart.
* Dryness of the throat and mouth.
* Impulsive behavior, emotional instability.
* Inability to concentrate or to listen to others.
* "Floating anxiety."
* Self-preoccupation.
* Emotional tension and alertness.
* Development of nervous habits (eye rolling, bruxism, teeth clenching).
* High-pitched, nervous laughter.
* Sweating.
* Loss of or excessive appetite.
* Increased smoking.
* Phobias, vague pains, unexplained symptoms.
* Sleep irregularities, including nightmares.
* Increased use of legally prescribed drugs (self-medication begins or increases).
* Pain in the neck or lower back, migraine headaches.
* Aphthous ulcers.
* Premenstrual tension or missed menstrual cycles.
* Factitial injuries (lip and/or cheek biting).
* Overpowering urge to cry or run and hide.
* Type A behavior as characterized by hurry, hostility, and impatience towards others; angry or excessive competitive pressures.†
* Inability to relax (guilty feelings when relaxing).
* Overwork; taking on excessive responsibilities.
* Resistance to change, suspicion, paranoia.
* Feelings of discouragement, indifference, and negativism.
* Postponement of patient contacts and phone calls.
* Delay or cancellation of vacation plans.
* Increase of illness susceptibility.

*These signs and symptoms often occur in clusters, may differ greatly from person to person, and are often vague.

†According to Rosenman, the type A behavior pattern is "an action-emotion complex exhibited by increasing numbers of individuals in their interaction with others and against opposition of time, persons, and things. It is not a personality typology but is a behavioral syndrome that is correlated with enhanced neurohormonal responses. It includes behavioral dispositions such as ambitiousness, aggressiveness, competitiveness and impatience; specific behaviors such as muscle tenseness, mental alertness, rapid and emphatic speech stylistics, and rapid pace of most activities; and emotional responses such as irritation, hostility and anger that is usually covert." There is considerable evidence that the type A behavior pattern is strongly related to the prevalence, incidence, and mortality rates of ischemic heart disease.

Identify and Anticipate Harmful Stressors

Merely identifying the source and nature of the stressors can have a therapeutic value, since we no longer have to unconsciously blame ourselves for our problems. Since we are really the best judges of ourselves, Selye urges each of us to learn how to carefully observe our own reactions to harmful stressors (we have just discussed these revealing physical and psychological body clues in Table 10–4). We often become so accustomed to stress that we are unaware of it. Still, its effects accumulate. Many dentists suffer the harmful effects of overstress even though they do not feel tense. Stress can damage the body even when a person does not feel frustrated or anxious. With practice, we can gradually develop instinctive feelings that tell us whether we are running above or below an acceptable personal stress level.

If we anticipate an especially stressful event in the future, it is possible to mentally rehearse a solution to our problem in advance. For example, if an individual who has recently quit smoking plans to attend a cocktail party where heavy smoking will occur, he can rehearse a strategy beforehand to prevent him from backsliding. He might plan to spend most of his time at the party with a nonsmoking friend who is supportive of his quit-smoking efforts. By identifying and anticipating a harmful stressor, he has markedly reduced the level of distress he will suffer in the presence of smokers. He is engaged in a direct-action form of coping and has mastered some level of the potential stress before it is encountered.

Use Multiple Active Strategies

Pines and Aronson showed that active strategies, especially those that are direct and multiple, are much more likely to change the source of stress than those that are passive (Fig 10–2). Passive strategies tend to emphasize withdrawal by means of avoidance, denial, or chemical escape. The abuse of alcohol, drugs, or nitrous oxide fits into this category. The frequency of these strategies is positively correlated to psychological burnout. Passive methods, called "false cures," provide only temporary relief, often have undesirable side effects, and fail to address the basic issue—resolution of the problem.

Develop a Positive Attitude and Life Philosophy

Active strategies are based on the development of positive attitudes toward the various events in our lives. Believing that emotions have a will of their own and cannot be controlled is a myth. Our emotions do not arise mysteriously from the subconscious or from the gut. Tension comes from

	Active	Passive
Direct	• CHANGING THE SOURCE OF THE STRESS • CONFRONTING SOURCE • ADOPTING A POSITIVE ATTITUDE	• IGNORING SOURCE OF THE STRESS • AVOIDING SOURCE • LEAVING
Indirect	• TALKING ABOUT THE SOURCE OF STRESS • CHANGING SELF • GETTING INVOLVED IN OTHER ACTIVITIES	• ALCOHOL OR DRUGS • GETTING ILL • COLLAPSING

Fig 10–2.—Stress-coping grid demonstrating four types of coping strategies used to counteract daily life stresses. (From Pines A.M., Aronson E.: *Burnout.* Schiller Park, Ill., MTI Teleprograms, Inc., 1980. Used by permission.)

factors we can gain control over. We can change our feelings by first changing our behavior, our thinking, and our attitudes. Active ways of coping often involve finding stress-reducing, enjoyable activities, hobbies, or other outside interests and developing a positive attitude and philosophy toward life. Attitude determines whether we perceive any experience as pleasant or unpleasant, and adopting the right one can convert a negative stress into a positive one.

When Godwin and coworkers questioned recent dental graduates concerning the methods they used to cope with excessive stress and anxiety, five methods were mentioned, but only two were common: sports, 47%; simple avoidance, 44%; family activities, 9%; religious activities, 8%; and alcohol or drugs, 8%. Most of these young dentists dealt with stress by passive, negatively oriented thinking and diversions instead of directly coping with them—a significant finding, because diversions do not address the underlying cause(s) of stress. Pines and Aronson stated the importance of using a variety of coping techniques rather than one strategy exclusively.

Likewise Dunlap and Stewart's 1981 to 1982 nationwide survey of 3,700 dentists indicated that a significant number had not learned effective stress-management skills. Notice the percentage of dentists who responded *always* or *frequently* to the following stress management strategies:

Get inadequate exercise	56%
Need to win at sports	34%

Feel distressed when decisions are questioned   33%
Dislike asking for help   29%
Have difficulty setting personal goals   27%
Fail to eat well-balanced meals once a day   24%

Time Management

Everyone is forced to spend time at a fixed rate because of the fact that it cannot be stockpiled. However, dentists continually complain that they are habitually out of time. Too much time can be a powerful stressor to the new dentist whose practice is not growing fast or to the established practitioner who is in one of those inevitable slumps. It is not uncommon for dentists to look at their watches eight times each half hour (128 times a day). This allows them to unconsciously reschedule their pace for the appointment. How we choose to use the time given to us is, to a great extent, within our control or determination. Management seminars frequently have addressed ways of effectively dealing with time, and Table 10–5 lists some of their recommendations.

TABLE 10–5.—SELECTED TECHNIQUES, DEVICES, AND METHODS TO AID IN TIME MANAGEMENT*

1. Set your *own* goals and objectives. Put them in writing so they become more concrete and specific. Look at them periodically.
2. At the start of each day, spend some time organizing your schedule. (One minute spent planning saves 20 minutes in execution.)
3. Assign priorities to each task and make a "To Do" list: "A" for the most urgent, "must-do" tasks, "B" for medium value, and "C" for nonurgent tasks (that may even go away if you wait long enough!).
4. Do not set unrealistic deadlines or goals for yourself or your subordinates.
5. Break down the overwhelming tasks into small, manageable steps or subgoals, which, when completed, give a sense of accomplishment and enthusiasm.
6. Complete tough tasks during your prime time.
7. Learn to recognize and overcome your own particular habits of time wasting.
8. Learn to say *no* to yourself and to others.
9. Do not strive for absolute perfection.
10. Ask yourself, "What is the best use of my time right now?"
11. Announce an agenda for meetings and stick to it. Set time limits.
12. Be sure employees know what is required of them. Include it in the office manual.
13. Try to handle paperwork only once.
14. Avoid postponing or making partial decisions unless the problems are very complex.
15. Read selectively or let others read for you. Let someone else get rid of the junk mail.
16. Delegate, delegate, delegate.
17. Use specialists and consultants liberally (get rid of your clinical frustrations by referral).
18. Without guilt, schedule daily "goof-off" time for relaxation.

*From Christen A.G., Harris N.O.: Office Safety: Future planning may prevent accidents. *Dent. Stud.* 60:32, 1981, and Katz C.A.: Managing to find the time. *Dent. Pract.* 2:26, 1981.

Developing Social Supports

Dr. Roy C. Menninger recently said that we give more attention to our lawn mowers than we give to the development of our personal relationships. One of the most effective methods of stress reduction is the ability to develop meaningful contact with others, including our peers. Whether in solo or group practice, it is relatively easy for dentists to become absolutely isolated socially. This can lead to bearing all problems and burdens alone, rather than sharing them with others. (However, it is certainly useless for groups of dentists to gather and reinforce their collective anxieties by exchanging unremitting tales of woe and predictions of doom!) Forrest stresses the importance of dentists learning to extend help to each other and to be more supportive socially. He reminds us that a combination of stress, life changes, and a lack of social support leads to suicide. We should be alert to suicidal warning signs in colleagues and, if we suspect such intentions, to convey our concern and willingness to help in a simple, direct, and compassionate way. Talk of suicide should be taken seriously. Other danger signals include a noticeable behavioral change, increasing indecisiveness and disorganization, withdrawal of interest in people, things, and activities, and sudden expressions of happiness.

An effective support group or network of relatives, friends, coworkers, neighbors, and community care givers provides us with concrete help and coping resources in dealing with our day-to-day problems. According to Caplan, a high level of group support offers many benefits to the individual, including the following:

1. Adds to his overall information base.

2. Helps him improve his own data collection.

3. Aids him in evaluating the situation and working out a sensible plan.

4. Assists him in implementing his plan, assessing its consequences, and replanning in line with the feedback of information.

5. Reminds him of his continuing identity, thereby bolstering his positive self-image.

6. Assures him that his discomforts in life are to be expected and, although burdensome, can usually be tolerated.

7. Maintains the hope that his efforts will produce some form of an ultimately successful outcome.

8. Protects against increased vulnerability to stress-related illnesses.

We each need to ask ourselves two questions: Is there anybody around us to whom we can *really* talk? If so, have we spoken to this person?

Dunlap and Stewart's large survey results indicate that dental office stress levels are reduced as more people become involved in a dental practice. There tends to be more sharing and stimulation, more camaraderie and exchange of ideas, and often more financial security in a group practice.

The support of a spouse is also of great importance to the dentist in reducing stress levels. If a dentist has experienced one of the three most stressful life events (death of a spouse, divorce, or marital separation), he or she has suffered a serious break or disruption in his or her social network. Marriage must be considered one of the most fundamental and intimate ties that can exist with another person. In fact, nonmarried people have higher mortality rates from almost every cause of death. Burke and Weir studied the reduced well-being in 189 professional men exposed to varying levels of job and life stress. They found that there was significantly lower incidence of negative well-being in highly stressed indviduals who received strong support from their wives, compared with those men similarly exposed to stress and unsupported by their wives. If social support and friendships are lacking at work, and marital problems exist at home, the dentist may be taxed beyond his ability to cope. Domestic difficulties may or may not have impact on the stresses of practice. However, the dentist may assume total responsibility for them with resultant feelings of guilt, followed by an overwhelming sense of hopelessness and profound depression.

Delegation and Cooperation

Our responsibilities as dentists have ethical and practical limits. However, we dentists are particularly prone to thinking that we are the only ones in the office who can assume responsibility and make decisions. This places us clearly in the untenable position of being omniscient and omnipresent—qualities better reserved for a deity. Although this thought may flatter our egos, it often places an unnecessary burden on us. Furthermore, it robs our employees of initiative and of the opportunity to grow professionally and personally. In actuality, the dentist, patients, and office workers need each other, and it is vital that their association is based on a spirit of mutual cooperation and trust. Cooperation is a dynamic social process in which the mutual benefits of working together far outweigh the disadvantages of competition.

According to Katz, "A general rule of thumb is not to spend your time and energy doing anything that could be done (legally, of course) by someone in the office—unless, of course, you want to do it." (*Dental Practice* 2:26, 1981.

If we are going to delegate responsibility, there are certain prerequisites that should be established (Table 10–6).

TABLE 10–6.—HOW TO EFFECTIVELY DELEGATE
RESPONSIBILITIES TO OTHERS*

- Form your own balanced, realistic, and clearly defined personal goals before delegating responsibilities to others.
- Make sure all staff members understand the office philosophy.
- Learn to accept your own human limitations of time, energy, and ability and also those of your office employees.
- Avoid making excessive demands of yourselves and of others; set realistic deadlines.
- Integrate the goals of the organization with those of subordinates.
- Learn from past mistakes and avoid negative self-talk and recrimination for past failures.
- Find out what's really going on in the office.
- Improve communication skills with subordinates and superiors; learn to listen without interrupting.
- Give employees challenging assignments.
- Learn how to tactfully supply negative and positive feedback, remembering that everyone needs time to perfect personal skills.
- Reward employees for high-quality performance.

*From Katz C.A.: Managing to find the time. *Dent. Pract.* 2:26, 1981, Troxler R.G.: Personal communication, 1982, and Troxler R.G., Cayton T.G.: Stress reduction for business and industrial employees, in Faber M.M., Reinhardt A.M. (eds.): *Promoting Health Through Risk Reduction.* New York, MacMillan Publishing Co., 1982, pp. 134–149.

Relaxation

WHY IS IT IMPORTANT?—Relaxation is important because it accomplishes the following:

1. Conserves productive energy that was previously wasted through tension and stress.

2. Can control nervous energy and focus it toward serving more useful purposes.

3. Often affects performance in a positive way because it increases energy and vitality, allowing a person's body to replenish its reserves.

4. Can help prepare an individual in advance to make better choices and more careful decisions when they are later required to respond under fire.

5. Helps the dentist who is skilled in stress management and relaxation discern more clearly the best strategy to employ in the office when being faced with an emotionally laden situation.

6. Leads to a relaxed appearance, which helps to inspire the patient's confidence and increases their trust level.

ELEMENTS OF RELAXATION.—Learning how to relax is an active strategy consisting of three elements: (1) recognizing tension, (2) releasing tension, and (3) relating relaxation methods to daily life routines.

DESTRESSING SKILLS.—Although there is no universal prescription for successful stress management, many enjoyable and rewarding activities often help to achieve a deep sense of physical and psychological relaxation and to sublimate our aggressive, hostile, and competitive energies. The possibilities are endless and diverse, but all have certain elements in common: they promote greater self-awareness, self-confidence, and self-esteem.

Destressing skills encompass a wide variety of activities from artistic, athletic, intellectual, physical, spiritual, and social areas. They may include the following:

- Progressive relaxation
- Meditation
- Biofeedback
- Yoga
- Autogenic training
- Imagery
- Self-hypnosis
- Exercise
- Proper diet/nutrition
- Value clarification

It is not possible in this chapter to discuss all of the above strategies, but there are many self-help books and articles from the popular press available to aid the reader.

While the above pursuits are all potentially beneficial, I believe activities that promote physical self-awareness through aerobic exercise are particularly important (e.g., walking, running/jogging, dancing, gymnastics, and group sports). One of the greatest natural (and legal) "highs" that one can experience is the sensation of a healthy body in motion. Our bodies were designed for activity, movement, grace, and rhythm. Emerson recognized this fact when he said, "First be a good animal" (see Christen and Cooper). Many individuals report that they have broken harmful habits (such as cigarette smoking) after embarking on a jogging or aerobic exercise program. The person who exercises faithfully is more apt to live prudently and be less inclined to engage in smoking, excessive drinking, overeating, or stress-causing behavior.

Physical activity can change the state of the mind, causing distinct and rapid changes in personality. When a sedentary, middle-aged, highly stressed man enters a long-term, strenuous physical conditioning program and continues to participate in it, he will gain a new sense of accomplishment, independence, and a sense of self-control. He is also likely to enjoy the exhilarating feeling of becoming more resolute, emotionally stable, and imaginative. Physical activity has been prescribed frequently in nonspecific ways as part of the therapeutic milieu of psychiatric rehabilitation programs. It is often used in the treatment of drug and alcohol abuse, juvenile delinquency, neurotic anxiety and specific situational phobias, and to provide psychological relief in postinfarct patients.

In a significant study of supervised physical activity in three metropolitan university settings, Heinzelmann and Bagley monitored 381 sedentary men (239 test and 142 control), ages 45 to 59, who were at risk in developing coronary heart disease. Many participants reported that they enjoyed having social support while they exercised and welcomed the opportunity to compare their own progress and level of fitness with the progress and fitness of others. An important finding was that the men's pattern of adherence to an exercise regimen was directly related to their wives' attitudes toward the program. Of the 143 men whose wives' attitudes were positive, 80% had good or excellent patterns of adherence. In contrast, only 40% of the 39 men whose wives' attitudes were neutral or negative had good or excellent patterns of adherence. In 1972, Durbeck and coworkers produced comparable results in the National Aeronautics and Space Administration–U.S. Public Health Service Health Evaluation and Enhancement Program (NASA-USPHS) with 237 exercising men from ages 35 to 55.

The conclusions of these studies are compared in Table 10–7. They clearly show how an exercise health program can reduce stress and promote healthful lifestyles.

TABLE 10–7.—HOW AN AEROBIC EXERCISE HEALTH PROGRAM HELPS PROMOTE PSYCHIC AND PHYSICAL HEALTH*

EXERCISE PROGRAM EFFECTS	UNIVERSITY STUDY (%)	NASA-USPHS STUDY (%)
Increased stamina	90	88
Feelings of better health	85	92
Weight reduction	67	61
Improved work performance	60	50
Decreased food consumption	48	48
Increased recreation	45	41
Reduced stress and tension	43	49
More positive work attitude	40	50
More adequate sleep and rest	37	30
Decreased smoking	20	15

*These findings are the results of two studies representing 476 exercising men. (From Christen A.G., Cooper K.H.: Strategic withdrawal from cigarette smoking. *CA Cancer J. Clinicians* 29:96, 1979. Used by permission.)

REFERENCES

Berkman L.F.: Social network analysis and coronary heart disease. *Adv. Cardiol.* 29:37, 1982.

Burke R.J., Weir T.: Marital helping relationships: The moderators between stress and well-being. *J. Psychol.* 95:121, 1977.

Caplan G.: Mastery of stress: Psychosocial aspects. *Am. J. Psychiatry* 138:413, 1981.

Christen A.G., Harris N.O. (eds.): Symposium on environmental protection in the dental operatory. *Dent. Clin. North Am.* 22:329, 1978.

Christen A.G., Cooper K.H.: Strategic withdrawal from cigarette smoking. *CA Cancer J. Clinicians* 29:96, 1979.

Christen A.G., Harris N.O.: Office safety: Future planning may prevent accidents. *Dent. Stud.* 60:32, 1981.

Cooper K.H.: *The Aerobics Way* (ed. 1). New York, M. Evans Co., 1977.

Cooper K.H., Christen A.G.: Dentist, "heal thyself": Modification of life style. *Dent. Clin. North Am.* 22:373, 1978.

Dunlap J.E., Stewart J.D.: Survey suggests less stress in group offices. *Dent. Economics* 72:46, 1982.

Durbeck D.C., Heinzelmann F., Schacker J., et al.: The National Aeronautics and Space Administration, U.S. Public Health Service Health Evaluation and Enhancement Program: Summary of results. *Am. J. Cardiol.* 30:784–790, 1972.

Eliot R.S., Forker A.D.: Emotional stress and cardiac disease. *J.A.M.A.* 236:2325, 1976.

Forrest W.R.: Stresses and self-destructive behavior of dentists. *Dent. Clin. North Am.* 22:361, 1978.

Gehrman R.: In search of serenity. *Dent. Management* 17:45, 1977.

Godwin W.C., Starks D.D., Green T.G., et al.: Identification of sources of stress in practice by recent dental graduates. *J. Dent. Educ.* 45:220–221, 1981.

Heinzelmann F., Bagley R.W.: Response to physical activity programs and their effects on health behavior. *Public Health Rep.* 85:905, 1970.

Holmes T.H., Rahe R.H.: The social readjustment rating scale. *J. Psychosom. Res.* 11:213, 1967.

Howard J.H., Cunningham D.A., Rechnitzer P.A., et al.: Stress in the job and career of a dentist. *J. Am. Dent. Assoc.* 93:630–636, 1976.

Ismail A.H., Trachtman L.E.: Jogging the imagination. *Psychol. Today* 6:79, 1973.

Jackson E., Mealiea W.L. Jr.: Stress management and personal satisfaction in dental practice. *Dent. Clin. North Am.* 21:559, 1977.

Katz C.A.: Reducing interpersonal stress in dental practice. *Dent. Clin. North Am.* 22:347, 1978.

Katz C.A.: Reducing stress: We never learned that people are more than just vehicles for the transportation of teeth. *Dent. Pract.* 1:50, 1980.

Katz C.A.: Serenity is not freedom from the storm, but peace amid the storm. *Dent. Pract.* 1:59, 1980.

Katz C.A.: Managing to find the time. *Dent. Pract.* 2:26, 1981.

Katz C.A.: *In Search of the Hardy Dentist.* Nexus Book VII, Dec. 21, 1981, Chapters 35–36.

Kobasa S.C.: Stressful life events, personality and health: An inquiry into hardiness. *J. Pers. Soc. Psychol.* 37:1, 1979.

Menninger R.C.: Address to the American College of Dentistry, Kansas City, Mo., Oct. 24, 1981.

Morse D.R.: Overcoming "practice stress" via medication and hypnosis. *Dent. Survey* 53:32, 1977.

Owen D.: The secret lives of dentists. *Harper's Mag.* 264:42, 1982.

Patrick P.K.S.: *Health Care Worker Burnout: What It Is, What To Do About It* (ed. 1). Chicago, Blue Cross Association, 1981.

Pines A.M., Aronson E.: *Burnout.* Schiller Park, Ill., MTI Teleprograms Inc., 1980.

Reeves J.B., Reeves H.C.: The interrelationship of work and recreation: A case study of the dentist. *Texas Dent. J.* 94:14, 1976.

Rosenman R.H.: Role of Type A behavior pattern in the pathogenesis and prognosis of ischemic heart disease. *Adv. Cardiol.* 29:77, 1982.

Selye H.: *Stress Without Distress* (ed. 1). Philadelphia, J.B. Lippincott Co., 1974.

Selye H., Cherry L.: On the real benefits of eustress. *Psychol. Today* 11:60, 1978.

Troxler R.G.: Personal communication, 1982.

Troxler R.G., Cayton T.G.: Stress reduction for business and industrial employees, in Faber M.M., Reinhardt A.M. (eds.): *Promoting Health Through Risk Reduction.* New York, MacMillan Publishing Co., 1982, pp. 134–149.

Chapter 11

A Dental Workplace Health and Safety Guide

Jeanne M. Stellman, Ph.D., and Jacqueline Messite, M.D.

MANY OF THE health hazards that can be found in the dental office, laboratory, and operatory can be eliminated with simple precautions and good practices. Dentists should take the time to "walk through" their office operations and procedures for the purpose of detecting problem areas that may affect their own health and safety as well as the health and safety of their staff and their patients. In addition, when procedural changes are being considered and/or newer materials and equipment are to be purchased for the office, the dentist should give some consideration to the potential hazards associated with them and see that the proper precautions are taken and adequate controls are in place before any changes are made. Dental staff should be made familiar with the potential hazards and instructed as to the necessary precautions to take.

To assist the dentist, the following guide is designed to help assess the adequacy of control of the dental workplace with regard to chemical hazards, infectious agents, noise, and other physical hazards.

Chemicals

Some General Practices Guidelines

For each of the chemical processes or products used, the following should be considered:

1. Do you know the generic name and potential toxic effects of each chemical ingredient?

2. Have you obtained material safety data sheets from the manufacturer?

3. Are all employees aware of proper handling practices and precautions?

4. Are in-service training sessions carried out at least annually?

5. Are you and your employees aware of signs and symptoms of inadvertent exposure?

6. Are records kept of the dates, quantities, and names of all chemicals used?

171

Specific Chemicals

Mercury

Mercury can enter the body by inhalation of vapors, absorption through the skin, and/or ingestion of particulates. Exposure can occur during preparation of amalgams, from persistent contamination of the office itself, which leads to a "background" level of mercury, or during procedures for removal of old amalgams and/or finishing of new restorations. In order to minimize potential exposures in your practice, do you observe the following guidelines?

1. Provide a well-ventilated work area for procedures involving mercury?

2. Use only tightly sealed capsules during amalgamation, preferably premeasured disposable ones?

3. Incorporate "no-touch" techniques for handling amalgam?

4. Limit the use of mercury to identified areas that meet standards for recommended practices?

5. Have seamless impervious flooring that is carried up the walls for at least 10 cm (covering)—not carpeting, which sequesters the mercury—in the dental operatories?

6. Provide work surface areas that are impervious to mercury contamination and lipped to contain and facilitate cleanup of accidental spills?

7. Know and provide training to employees on appropriate cleanup of accidental spills? (Washing hands with a weak solution of sodium thiosulfate will remove mercury.)

8. Have an accessible supply of a polysulfide compound for use in cleanup?

9. Store mercury in unbreakable, sealed containers in a cool area?

10. Routinely salvage and store in sealed containers all amalgam scraps?

11. Monitor the air to ascertain that there is at least minimal compliance with the federal mercury vapor in air standard of 0.10 mg/m^3 (average per 8-hour day)? (It would be preferable to keep the mercury level in the air below the National Institute for Occupational Safety and Health and American Dental Association recommended level of 0.05 mg/m^3 (average per 8-hour day.)

12. For employees for whom a significant exposure to mercury is possible, do you (a) carry out biological assays (e.g., urinary mercury) on employees at risk of exposure and repeat assays on positive findings and (b) provide these employees with passive dosimeters for mercury?

Anesthetic Gases

Anesthetic gases can pollute the dental environment during administration of these gases and from patient exhalation. Pollution can extend beyond the operatory to office, waiting rooms, and even to the closets, particularly when air conditioning systems recirculate the air. Have you minimized potential exposure by observing the following?

1. Installing scavenging equipment on nasal masks? (This is very useful, but may not provide total control.)

2. Routinely checking for leakage in the anesthesia/analgesia machinery including the following?

- Wall connectors
- Hose connectors
- Compression fittings
- Gaskets and seals
- Threading in flowmeter tubes

This check should include turning off all cylinder valves and flowmeters overnight and reading pressure in the morning. (More than 10% loss under normal working pressure indicates leakage.)

3. Replacing all defective parts and contracting for professional preventive maintenance of machinery at least semiannually?

4. Venting the suction machine to an outside area away from all air intake sources to avoid recirculation of contaminated air?

5. Limiting patient speech after anesthesia/analgesia?

6. Establishing an air-monitoring program, including an internal assessment and repeated monitoring every 4 months?

7. Establishing a protocol for finding and eliminating leaks should air levels in excess of 50 ppm be measured?

Other Chemicals

ASBESTOS.—This toxic, cancer-causing mineral has been a component of powder for periodontal dressings and in liners for casting rings and crucibles. All unnecessary exposure to this dust and contamination of work areas should be avoided.

1. Do you know the asbestos content of your periodontal packs and/or casting ring and crucible liners?

2. Are all personnel informed and trained about potential hazards to asbestos?

3. Have you sought nonasbestos-containing substitutes?

BERYLLIUM.—If beryllium alloys are being used in your facility, have you observed the following?

1. Have the operations been evaluated for the degree of exposure, and is there adequate ventilation to ensure control?

2. Is your staff informed of its toxicity and proper procedures for use?

Ethylene oxide (EtO).—If EtO sterilization is used in your practice, the following guidelines should be considered:

1. Are the sterilizers exhausted to a safe outdoor location?

2. Do they have interlocks to prevent opening when they are being used?

3. Are work procedures and protective clothing adequate to protect personnel from skin or eye contact?

4. Because EtO is highly flammable, have measures been taken to keep the use of EtO away from all sources of ignition?

Methacrylate.—The following should be considered in the use of methacrylate:

1. Is there adequate ventilation to prevent excessive buildup of vapors?

2. Have measures been taken to keep skin contact to a minimum?

Infection Control

Hepatitis B, herpes, and other infections can be contracted from the close contact between patient and dentist, often through contact with saliva and blood. To avoid this, the following protective measures should be taken:

1. Do you take a complete health history of your patients, with an update each visit?

2. Do you use a rubber dam to limit the spread of aerosolized saliva?

3. Do you use surgical gloves to stop infections from entering abraded or nicked skin?

4. Do you wear a face mask while working on the patient?

5. Do you buy handpieces and air-water syringes that can be heat sterilized?

6. Are all dental instruments routinely and regularly sterilized?

7. Are disposable syringes and needles used and disposed of in closed containers?

8. Do you routinely have your patient rinse his/her mouth prior to beginning the session?

9. Are all uniforms and work clothes removed at work and laundered professionally to avoid contaminating home environments?

Radiation

Ionizing Radiation

The basic assumption is that all personnel recognize the need for judicious use of radiographic examination and for minimizing all unavoidable exposures. In addition, the following should be considered:

1. Are you fully aware of the latest techniques and requirements for the safe use of radiation?

2. Are only films rated Speed Group "D" or faster used?

3. Is the x-ray beam filtered to eliminate unnecessary wavelengths and to meet state and federal requirements? Do you minimize both the time and amperage needed to achieve effective results?

4. Do you provide patients with a leaded apron?

5. Do you always avoid holding the film in place for a patient and use x-ray holders or other methods instead?

6. Is your examination area arranged to permit you to stand at least 6 feet from the patient and outside the path of the beam when the equipment is operating?

7. If your workload is greater than 30 mamp per week, do you have an adequately screened and shielded area?

8. Do you have your office inspected periodically by state officials or other qualified experts to ensure that all equipment and shielding are effectively maintained? (Have you considered personal dosimeter measurements for you and your staff to assure control?)

9. Is your dark room well maintained, and are procedures and chemicals adequate to avoid ruining films, necessitating reradiation?

Nonionizing Radiation

1. Are these sources regularly maintained and serviced by the supplier?

2. Are all sources of ultraviolet radiation located or shielded so that eye exposure and contact are minimized?

Ears, Eyes, and Musculoskeletal Strains

1. Do you and your staff wear earplugs that allow normal sounds and speech to be transmitted, but block high frequency-intensity sounds?

2. Do you wear safety glasses to protect against flying debris and infectious agents, such as hepatitis B virus, which can penetrate the membranes of the eye?

3. Do you and your employees have stools with adjustable height, a broad stable base, firmly padded seat, a back support that can be shifted to support the side or abdomen, and freely rolling casters with ease of mobility?

4. Is there a foot rest for working positions where the operator cannot comfortably reach the floor?

5. Does your work position allow you to assume biomechanically appropriate postures including the following?

* Elbows close to side with the patient height adjusted for this position.
* Spine straight either when sitting or standing, with shoulders relaxed.
* Eyes directed downward, but neck not bent.

Safety

1. Are medical gas cylinders securely fastened to prevent falling and possible valve damage?

2. Is smoking prohibited in anesthetizing locations?

3. Are all flammable chemicals and films properly stored and labeled?

4. Is all electrical equipment properly grounded?

5. Have frayed cords or loose plugs been replaced?

6. Is there a smoke detector?

Stress

To avoid stress, do you practice the following?

1. Review scheduling practices to eliminate as much overscheduling as possible?

2. Have periodic dentist-dental staff meetings to discuss problem areas?

Appendix

Available Resources and Assistance

There are many governmental agencies that can help the dental professional by answering questions and providing screening or monitoring services. Dentists should not fear dealing with these agencies. At the very least, they can help you to evaluate your offices and prevent occupational health and safety hazards for you and your staff. This is especially important, because there is a federal law covering occupational safety and health for all workers requiring employers, including dentists, to provide safe and healthful workplaces for their employees. In addition, in some states and municipalities* there are the Workers' Right to Know laws, requiring employers to provide to their employees, on request, information including their work exposures.

To carry out your responsibilities under these various laws, you need to be familiar with your work operations and the materials used in your offices and have readily available information about the toxicity of the materials and the degree of exposure to them. Resources are available to assist the dentist and dental personnel in obtaining information and services to evaluate occupational health safety problems in their offices and clinics. This section identifies various official and nonofficial agencies to which health professionals can turn for advice on occupational health and safety. The list is by no means a complete one. In addition to those listed here, dentists should familiarize themselves with their local poison control centers, which have information on the toxicity of various chemical and pharmaceutical agents. Also, various insurance companies, particularly those involved with workers' compensation claims, offer to their clients materials and services including industrial hygiene survey assistance. A number of voluntary organizations such as the American Conference of Governmental Industrial Hygienists, American Industrial Hygiene Association, American Occupational Medical Association, American Academy of Occupational Medicine, etc., can provide information and educational materials and can suggest the

---

*California; Connecticut; Maine; Michigan; New York; Wisconsin; West Virginia; Cincinnati, Ohio; Pennsauken, N.J.; Philadelphia, Pa.; and San Diego, Calif.

availability of consultants to evaluate dental premises. Dentists and dental personnel should become familiar with the resources that are available in their areas.

PL 91–596: Occupational Safety and Health Act.

With the passage of the Occupational Safety and Health Act of 1970, two major federal agencies involved in the evaluation of occupational safety and health problems were created. These are the Occupational Safety and Health Administration in the Department of Labor and the National Institute for Occupational Safety and Health in the Department of Health and Human Services.

The National Institute for Occupational Safety and Health (NIOSH) has the following responsibilities:

1. To develop criteria for the establishment of national occupational safety and health standards.

2. To collect and analyze records and statistics on occupational safety and health necessary for promulgation of new or improved mandatory occupational safety and health standards.

3. To develop criteria for dealing with toxic materials and harmful physical agents, indicating safe exposure levels for workers for various periods of time, in consultation with the Department of Labor.

4. To make toxicity determinations on request by employer or employee groups.

5. To publish an annual listing of all known toxic substances and the concentrations at which such toxicity is known to occur.

The NIOSH can provide the dentists and dental staff with information about the toxic substances they use and will perform, on written request, health hazard evaluations of the work operations. There are ten regional offices of NIOSH.

NIOSH Regional Offices

Region I (Massachusetts, Connecticut, Maine, New Hampshire, Rhode Island, Vermont):
DHHS,* Government Center (J.F.K. Federal Bldg.)
Boston, MA 02203
617-223-6668

---

*Department of Health and Human Services.

Region II (New York, New Jersey, Puerto Rico, Virgin Islands):
DHHS, Jacob Javits Federal Bldg.
26 Federal Plaza
New York, NY 10278
212-264-2485

Region III (Delaware, District of Columbia, Maryland, Pennsylvania,
Virginia, West Virginia):
DHHS, P.O. Box 13716
Philadelphia, PA 19101
215-596-6716

Region IV (Alabama, Florida, Georgia, Kentucky, Mississippi, North
Carolina, South Carolina, Tennessee):
DHHS, DPHS†
101 Marietta Tower, Suite 1007
Atlanta, GA 30303
404-221-2396

Region V (Illinois, Indiana, Michigan, Minnesota, Ohio, Wisconsin):
DHHS
300 S. Wacker Dr., 33rd Floor
Chicago, IL 60606
312-886-3881

Region VI (Arkansas, Louisiana, New Mexico, Oklahoma, Texas):
DHHS
1200 Main Tower Bldg., Room 1700-A
Dallas, TX 75202
214-767-3916

Region VII (Iowa, Kansas, Missouri, Nebraska):
DHHS
601 E. 12th St.
Kansas City, MO 64106
816-374-5332

Region VIII (Colorado, Montana, North Dakota, South Dakota, Utah,
Wyoming):
DHHS/PHS‡/Prevention
Denver, CO 80294
303-837-3979

---

†Department of Public Health Service.
‡Public Health Service.

Region IX (American Samoa, Arizona, California, Commonwealth of the
  Northern Marianas, Guam, Hawaii, Nevada, Trust Territory of the
  Pacific Islands):
DHHS
50 United Nations Plaza
San Francisco, CA 94102
415-556-3781

Region X (Alaska, Idaho, Oregon, Washington):
DHHS
1321 Second Ave. (Arcade Plaza Bldg.)
Seattle, WA 98101
206-442-0530

OSHA Responsibilities

The Occupational Safety and Health Administration (OSHA) has the following responsibilities:

1. To promulgate, modify, and improve mandatory occupational safety and health standards.

2. To enforce the Act, with authority to enter factories and other workplace areas to conduct inspections and investigations of working conditions, equipment, and materials, and to issue citations and impose penalties.

3. To prescribe regulations requiring employers to maintain accurate records and reports concerning work-related injury, illness, and death, employee exposure to potentially toxic substances or other such records as considered appropriate, in cooperation with the DHHS.

4. To develop and maintain a system of collecting, compiling, and analyzing occupational safety and health statistics, in consultation with the DHHS.

5. To establish and supervise programs for the education and training of employee and employer personnel in the recognition, avoidance, and prevention of unsafe or unhealthful working conditions covered by the Act, in consultation with the DHHS.

6. To conduct directly or by grants and contracts educational and training programs aimed at providing an adequate supply of qualified personnel to carry out the purposes of the Act and to conduct information programs on the importance of and proper use of adequate safety and health equipment.

The OSHA can provide dental staff with information on health and safety matters in the offices and clinics and on the applicable existing OSHA standards for them. There are ten regional offices under the U.S. Department of Labor as follows:

OSHA Regional Offices

Region I (Connecticut, Maine, Massachusetts, New Hampshire, Rhode Island, Vermont):
16-18 North St.
1 Dock Square, Fourth Floor
Boston, MA 02109
617-223-6710

Region II (New York, New Jersey, Puerto Rico, Virgin Islands):
Room 3445, 1 Astor Plaza
1515 Broadway
New York, NY 10036
212-944-3426

Region III (Delaware, District of Columbia, Maryland, Pennsylvania, Virginia, West Virginia):
Gateway Blvd., Suite 2100
3535 Market St.
Philadelphia, PA 19104
215-596-1201

Region IV (Alabama, Florida, Georgia, Kentucky, Mississippi, North Carolina, South Carolina, Tennessee):
1375 Peachtree St. N.E.
Suite 587
Atlanta, GA 30367

Region V (Illinois, Indiana, Michigan, Minnesota, Ohio, Wisconsin):
230 S. Dearborn St.
32nd Floor, Room 3230
Chicago, IL 60604
312-353-2220

Region VI (Arkansas, Louisiana, New Mexico, Oklahoma, Texas):
555 Griffin Square, Room 602
Dallas, TX 75202
214-767-4731

Region VII (Iowa, Kansas, Missouri, Nebraska):
911 Walnut St., Room 3000
Kansas City, MO 64106
816-374-5861

Region VIII (Colorado, Montana, North Dakota, South Dakota, Utah, Wyoming):
Federal Bldg., Room 1554
1961 Stout St.
Denver, CO 80294
303-837-5285

Region IX (California, Arizona, Nevada, Hawaii, Guam, American Samoa, Trust Territory of the Pacific Islands):
450 Golden Gate Ave., Box 36017
San Francisco, CA 94102
415-556-0584

Region X (Alaska, Idaho, Oregon, Washington):
Federal Office Bldg., Room 6003
909 First Ave.
Seattle, WA 98174
206-442-5930

States With Approved OSHA Plans

The following states, under PL 91-596, have approved plans regarding enforcement activities:

Alaska
Edmund N. Orbeck, Commissioner
Alaska Dept. of Labor
P.O. Box 1149
Juneau, AK 99811
907-465-2700

Arizona
Larry Etchechury, Director
Division of Occupational Safety & Health
Industrial Commission of Arizona
P.O. Box 19070
Phoenix, AZ 85005
602-255-5795

California
Donald Vial, Director
California Dept. of Industrial Relations
525 Golden Gate Ave.
San Francisco, CA 94102
415-557-3356

Connecticut   P. Joseph Peraro, Commissioner (public employees only)
Connecticut Dept. of Labor
200 Folly Brook Blvd.
Wethersfield, CT 06109
203-566-5123

Hawaii   Joshua C. Agsalud, Director
Hawaii Dept. of Labor & Industrial Relations
825 Mililani St.
Honolulu, HI 96813
808-548-3150

Indiana   Howard E. Williams, Commissioner
Indiana Division of Labor
1013 State Office Bldg.
100 North Senate Ave.
Indianapolis, IN 46204
317-232-2663

Iowa   Allen J. Meier, Commissioner
Iowa Bureau of Labor
State House
307 E. Seventh St.
Des Moines, IA 50319
515-281-3447

Kentucky   John Calhoun Wells, Commissioner
Kentucky Dept. of Labor
U.S. Highway 127 S.
Frankfort, KY 40601
502-564-3070
FTS: 351-3070

Maryland   Harvey A. Epstein, Commissioner
Maryland Division of Labor & Industry
Dept. of Licensing & Regulation
203 E. Baltimore St.
Baltimore, MD 21202
301-659-4176

Michigan   William Long, Director
Michigan Dept. of Labor
7150 Harris Dr., Box 30015
Lansing, MI 48909
517-373-9600

Dr. Bailus Walker, Director
Michigan Dept. of Public Health
3500 N. Logan St., Box 30035
Lansing, MI 48909
517-373-1320

Minnesota   Russell B. Swanson, Commissioner
                   Minnesota Dept. of Labor & Industry
                   444 Lafayette Rd.
                   St. Paul, MN 55101
                   612-296-2342

Nevada   Alan Traenkner, Director
                   Nevada Dept. of Occupational Safety & Health
                   515 E. Musser St.
                   Carson City, NV 89714
                   702-885-5240

New Mexico   Russell Rhoades, Director
                   New Mexico Occupational Health & Safety Bureau
                   Health & Environment Dept.
                   1480 St. Francis Dr.
                   Santa Fe, NM 87504-0968
                   505-827-5273

North Carolina   John C. Brooks, Commissioner
                   North Carolina Dept. of Labor
                   4 W. Edenton St.
                   Raleigh, NC 27601
                   919-733-7166

Oregon   Roy G. Green, Director
                   Workers' Compensation Dept.
                   Labor & Industries Bldg.
                   Salem, OR 97310
                   503-378-3304

Puerto Rico   Pedro Barez Rosario
                   Secretary of Labor & Human Resources
                   Puerto Rico Dept. of Labor
                   Prudencio Rivera Martinez Bldg.
                   505 Munoz Rivera Ave.
                   Hato Rey, PR 00918
                   809-754-2119
                              2120
                              2121
                              2122

South Carolina	Edgar L. McGowan, Commissioner South Carolina Dept. of Labor 3600 Forest Dr. P.O. Box 11329 Columbia, SC 29211 803-758-2851 758-3080
Tennessee	J.B. Richesin, Jr., Commissioner Tennessee Dept. of Labor ATTN: Robert Taylor 501 Union Bldg. Suite "A" – Second Floor Nashville, TN 37219 615-741-2582
Utah	Walter T. Axelgard, Commissioner Utah Industrial Commission 350 E. Fifth S. Salt Lake City, UT 84111 801-533-4415
Vermont	Jeffrey L. Amestoy, Commissioner Vermont Dept. of Labor & Industry 118 State St. Montpelier, VT 05602 FTS-832-2286 802-828-2765
Virgin Islands	Richard Upson, Commissioner of Labor Government of Virgin Islands Box 890 Christiansted St. Croix, VI 00820 809-773-1994
Virginia	Azie Taylor Morton, Commissioner Virginia Dept. of Labor & Industry P.O. Box 12064 Richmond, VA 23241-0064 804-786-2376 Dr. James B. Kenley, Commissioner Virginia Dept. of Health James Madison Bldg. 109 Governor St. Richmond, VA 23219 FTS-936-4265

Washington   Samuel Kinville, Director
Washington Dept. of Labor & Industries
General Administration Bldg.
Room 334 – AX-31
Olympia, WA 98504
206-753-6307

Wyoming   Donald Owsley, Administrator
Dept. of Occupational Safety & Health
604 East 25th St.
Cheyenne, WY 82002
307-777-7786
    777-7787

The following states under PL91-596 provide consultative services only:

Alabama   Assistant Commissioner
Alabama State Dept. of Labor
600 Administration Bldg.
64 North Union St.
Montgomery, AL 36130
205-832-6270

American Samoa   Director
Dept. of Manpower Resources
Government of American Samoa
Pago Pago, AS 96920

Arkansas   Director
Dept. of Labor
1022 High St.
Little Rock, AR 72202
501-371-3024

Colorado   Executive Director
Dept. of Labor & Employment
251 E. 12th Ave.
Denver, CO 80203
303-866-2782

All paperwork to:

Director
Division of Labor
State Centennial Bldg.
1313 Sherman St., Room 314
Denver, CO 80203
303-866-2782

Delaware	Chief Dept. of Labor 820 N. French St. State Office Bldg. – Sixth Floor Wilmington, DE 19801 302-571-2710
District of Columbia	Director of Industrial Safety Government of the District of Columbia Office of Occupational Safety & Health 2900 Newton St. N.E. Washington, DC 20018 202-832-1230
	Mailing address:
	950 Upsur St. N.W. Washington, DC 20011 202-576-7100
Florida	Director Division of Labor Ashley Bldg., Room 200 1321 Executive Center Dr. E. Tallahassee, FL 32301 904-488-7396
Georgia	Commissioner Dept. of Labor State Labor Bldg. Atlanta, GA 30334
Guam	Director, Dept. of Labor Government of Guam 23548 Guam Main Facility Agana, GU 96921 671-772-6291
Idaho	Director Dept. of Labor Room 400, State House 317 Main St. Boise, ID 83720 208-334-3950

Illinois	Director Dept. of Labor 910 S. Michigan Ave. Chicago, IL 60605 312-793-2800
	Chairman Illinois Industrial Commission 160 N. LaSalle St., Room 1200 Chicago, IL 60601 312-793-6550
Kansas	Secretary Dept. of Human Resources 401 Topeka Ave. Topeka, KS 66603 913-296-7474
Louisiana	Secretary Louisiana Dept. of Labor 1045 State Land & National Resource Bldg. Baton Rouge, LA 70801 504-389-5314
Mariana Islands	Chief Labor Administrator Dept. of Commerce & Labor Comm. of the N. Mariana Islands Saipan, Mariana Islands 96950 808-546-3157
Maine	Commissioner Maine Comm. of Manpower Affairs 20 Union St. Augusta, ME 04330 207-289-3814
Massachusetts	Commissioner Mass. Dept. of Labor & Industry 100 Cambridge St. Boston, MA 02202 617-727-3454
Mississippi	Director of Occupational Safety & Health 2423 N. State St. P.O. Box 1700 Jackson, MS 39205 601-982-6315

Montana	Director Montana Dept. of Labor, Workmen's Comp. Div. 815 Front St. Helena, MT 59601 402-449-2047
Nebraska	Commissioner Dept. of Labor 550–50 16th St. Lincoln, NE 68509 402-475-8451
New Hampshire	Director Occupational Health Services Bureau 1 Pillsbury St. Concord, NH 03301 603-271-2281
New Jersey	Commissioner, Labor/Industry Labor & Industry Bldg. John Fitch Plaza Trenton, NJ 08625 609-292-2323
New York	Industrial Commissioner Dept. of Labor State Campus Bldg. #22 Albany, NY 12248 518-457-2741
North Dakota	Chairman N.D. Workmen's Comp. Bureau Highway 83, Route 1 Bismarck, ND 58501 701-255-4011
Ohio	Director Division of Occupational Safety & Health Dept. of Industrial Relations 2323 W. Fifth Ave. Columbus, OH 43204 614-466-4124
Oklahoma	Commissioner Oklahoma Dept. of Labor State Capitol, Room 118 Oklahoma City, OK 73109 405-521-2461

Pennsylvania   Secretary
                  Dept. of Labor & Industry
                  1700 Labor & Industry Bldg.
                  Harrisburg, PA 17120
                  717-787-3157

                  Secretary
                  Environmental Resources
                  519 S. Office Bldg.
                  Harrisburg, PA 17119
                  717-787-2814

Rhode Island   Director
                  R.I. Division of Occupational Safety/Dept. of Labor
                  220 Elmwood Ave.
                  Providence, R.I. 02908
                  401-277-2500

South Dakota   Secretary
                  Dept. of Health
                  Joe Foss Bldg.
                  Pierre, SD 57501
                  FTS 8-605-733-3361

Texas   Director
                  Texas State Dept. of Health & Safety
                  1100 W. 49th St.
                  Austin, TX 78756
                  521-397-5721, ext. 275

                  All paperwork to:

                  1100 W. 49th St.
                  Austin, TX 78756

Trust Territory   (see Mariana Islands)
  of the Pacific

West Virginia   Director
                  West Virginia Dept. of Labor
                  State Capitol
                  Charleston, WV 25305
                  304-348-2971

Acting Commissioner
West Virginia Dept. of Labor
State Capitol
Charleston, WV 25305
304-348-7890

Wisconsin   Secretary
Dept. of Industry, Labor & Human Relations
201 E. Washington Ave.
P.O. Box 7946
Madison, WI 53707

Educational Resource Centers

The following educational resource centers provide training in all occupational and environmental disciplines in the field and in research. These centers can also provide the dental professional with valuable information.

Alabama Educational Resource Center
University of Alabama at Birmingham
School of Public Health
Medical Center, University Station
Birmingham, AL 35294
205-934-6080
FTS 8-229-1000
Dr. Vernon E. Rose, Dr. P.H., Director

Arizona Educational Resource Center
University of Arizona
Arizona Health Sciences Center
1145 N. Warren – ACOSH
Tuscon, AZ 85724
602-626-6835
Herbert K. Abrams, M.D., Director

California Educational Resource Center – Northern
University of California, Berkeley
206 Earl Warren Hall
Berkeley, CA 94720
415-642-0761
Robert C. Spear, Ph.D., Director

California Educational Resource Center – Southern
University of California, Irvine
Dept. of Community & Environmental Medicine
Irvine, CA 91717
714-833-6269
B. Dwight Culver, M.D., Director

Cincinnati Educational Resource Center
University of Cincinnati
Institute of Environmental Health
3223 Eden Ave.
Cincinnati, OH 45267
513-872-5701
Raymond S. Suskind, M.D., Director

Harvard Educational Resource Center
Dept. of Environmental Health Sciences
Harvard School of Public Health
665 Huntington Ave.
Boston, MA 02115
617-732-1260
David Wegman, M.D., Director

Illinois Educational Resource Center
University of Illinois
School of Public Health
P.O. Box 6998
Chicago, IL 60680
312-996-2591
Bertram W. Carnow, M.D., Director

Johns Hopkins Educational Resource Center
Johns Hopkins University
School of Hygiene & Public Health
615 N. Wolfe St.
Baltimore, MD 21205
301-955-3900
    955-3720
Morton Corn, M.D., Director

Michigan Educational Resource Center
University of Michigan
Dept. of Industrial & Operations Engineering
2260 S.G. Brown Laboratory
Ann Arbor, MI 48109
313-763-2245
FTS 8-963-2245
Don B. Chaffin, Ph.D., Director

Minnesota Educational Resource Center
University of Minnesota
School of Public Health
1162 Mayo Memorial
420 Delaware St. S.E.
Minneapolis, MN 55455
612-221-8770
Robert O. Mulhausen, M.D., Director

New York/New Jersey Educational Resource Center
Mt. Sinai School of Medicine
1 Gustave Levy Pl.
New York, NY 10029
212-650-6174
Irving J. Selikoff, M.D., Director

North Carolina Educational Resource Center
109 Conner Dr.
Professional Village
346 A, Suite 1101
Chapel Hill, NC 27514
919-962-2101
David S. Fraser, Sc.D., Director

Texas Educational Resource Center
The University of Texas Health Science Center at Houston
School of Public Health
P.O. Box 20186
Houston, TX 77025
713-792-7450
Dr. Fairchild, Acting Director

Utah Educational Resource Center
Rocky Mountain Center for Occupational & Environmental Health
University of Utah Medical Center
DFCM, Room BC 106
Salt Lake City, UT 84132
801-581-8719
William N. Rom, M.D., Director

Washington Educational Resource Center
University of Washington
Dept. of Environmental Health SC-34
Seattle, WA 98195
206-543-4383
John T. Wilson, Jr., M.D., Director

Standards Governing Use of Toxic Substances in Dental Practice*

	OSHA† EXISTING STANDARD	NIOSH‡ RECOMMENDED STANDARD	ACGIH§ THRESHOLD LIMIT VALUE
Mercury as Hg	0.1 mg/m³‖	0.05 mg/m³	0.05 mg/m³
Waste anesthetic gases	...		...
Nitrous oxide	...	25 ppm ¶**	...
Halogenated agents (halothane, methoxyflurane, etc.)	...	2 ppm (1-hr ceiling)	...
Asbestos	2 fibers/cc††	0.1 fiber/cc	0.5 fiber/cc (amosite)
	10 fibers/cc ceiling	0.5 fiber/cc (15-min intervals)	0.2 fiber/cc (crocidolite)
	0.5 fibers/cc (proposed)		2.0 fibers/cc (chrysotile and other forms)
	5 fibers/cc ceiling (proposed)		
Methyl methacrylate (510 mg/m³)	100 ppm		100 ppm (410 mg/m³)
			125 ppm (STEL)‡‡
Ethylene oxide	50 ppm		10 ppm (20 mg/m³)
	1 ppm (proposed)		1 ppm (2 mg/m³) (intended change)

*Values are for 8 hr/day (OSHA and ACGIH) or 10 hr/day, 40 hr/wk, unless stated as ceiling or STEL value.
†Occupational Safety and Health Administration.
‡National Institute for Occupational Safety and Health.
§American Conference of Governmental Industrial Hygienists.
‖Milligrams per cubic meter of air.
¶Parts per million parts of air.
**According to NIOSH publication 77-140, *Criteria Document on Waste Anesthetic Gases*, exposure levels for nitrous oxide of 50 ppm and less are achievable with current control technology in dental offices.
††Fibers> 5 μm in length.
‡‡Short-term exposure limit.

Index

197

aerosols and, 32
Lasix: and hearing loss, 128–129
Lathe: hazards of, 92
Laws: Workers' Right to Know, 177
Leg problems, 137
Leukemia: and ethylene oxide, 10
Leukocyte counts: and radiation
    exposure, 110
Light
  Castle Panovision, 141
  fluorescent, 143
  halide, 141–142
  probe, Elipar, 97
  visible light radiation, 13, 97
Lighting
  office, 141–143
  task-area, 142–143
Lips
  chancres on, 60
  in gonorrhea, 62
Liquids: flammable, precautions for,
    101
Liver
  cancer (*see* Cancer, liver)
  disease after exposure to anesthetic
    gases, 8, 82, 83, 87
Lordosis, 137, 139, 140
Low back pain, 139
Lung
  beryllium and, 12
  cancer (*see* Cancer, lung)
Lupus erythematosus: discoid, and
    dental operating lights, 143
Lysine: and herpes simplex, 48

M

Machines: problems with, 134–135
Malpractice insurance, 145
Mantoux test, 40
Manual: office administrative, 145
Masks: face, 27–28
Mèniére's disease, 131
Mercurialism: chronic, symptoms of,
    72–73
Mercury, 10–11, 71–78, 136
  biologic evaluations, 75
  blood levels, 72
  contamination
    office design and, 75

sources of, 74
exposure, 74
health and safety guidelines, 172
historical background, 71
hygiene, dental, 72–77
hypersensitivity, 10–11
monitoring
  devices, 74–75
  office, 74
  personal, 74–75
physical properties, 72
pregnancy and, 11
problem
  current, 71–73
  extent of, 73
spill cleanup kits, 77
storage, 75–76
urinary values, 72
vapor, ambient, threshold limit value
    for, 72
Mesotheliomas
  asbestos causing, airborne, 9
  ethylene oxide causing, 10
Metals: molten, ultraviolet radiation
    from, 96–97
Methacrylate, 9, 104, 105–106
  health and safety guidelines, 174
Methyl
  alcohol, 101, 104
  ethyl ketone, 101
  methacrylate, 9, 104, 105–106
  health and safety guidelines, 174
Methylene chloride, 104
MHA-TP, 61
Miconazole
  in candidiasis, 43
  in dermatophytosis, 43
Microdentistry, 142
Microhemagglutination *T. pallidum*
    test, 61
Microscopy: electron, in herpes
    simplex, 47
Microwave radiation, 99
Mineral dusts, 9
Molten metals: ultraviolet radiation
    from, 96–97
Monitoring
  equipment, nitrous oxide trace gas,
    85
  mercury (*see* Mercury, monitoring)